THE

LOST

TRIBE

**Stories from survivors of Cauda
Equina Syndrome**

FOREWORD
by
Mr Munawar Mecci
Consultant Spinal Cord Injuries
Golden Jubilee SCI Centre, James
Cook University Hospital

It wasn't until 2012 that the Department of Health recognised the recommendation made by the Spinal Cord Injury Clinical Reference Group, that patients with Cauda Equina Syndrome should be treated by specialist healthcare staff in spinal cord injury centres. This recommendation was approved by the Trauma Programme of Care Board and all local NHS organizations were to be made aware of the recommendation. And yet, in 2015, when I was shown this information by former CES patient Annie Glover, at a conference of the Multidisciplinary Association for Spinal Cord Injury Professionals, I was still not aware of this very important group of patients that needed our care.

I started to look at the services we provided at the Golden Jubilee Spinal Cord Injuries Centre and found that CES patients are what, I describe as *THE LOST TRIBE*. They were incontinent of bladder and bowel and imbibed with shame, not having the courage to venture out. They were in fact, self-isolating. There was no socializing, no parties, no going to the pub or on holidays. Relationships were breaking down, jobs were lost. Everything was lost. They were marooned with no hope of rescue in sight.

We clearly needed to get our own house in order with respect to these patients. Firstly, we found that over a ten-year period (2006-16), out of 84 patients with a diagnosis of CES, who had been operated on, only 7 of them were under my care.

We needed one service, under one roof, providing holistic care for this group. We also needed a pathway which identifies patients who develop CES and ensures early referral to the regional spinal cord injuries centre. And we needed to make sure the patient no longer feels the condition is only in their mind, which many do when CES is not taken seriously enough.

In 2016 we established the first clinic with the holistic, clearly identified pathway needed, provided under one roof. Here, there is no such thing as a brief admission for these patients. They are admitted and supported for as long as it takes. They should be treated the same as any spinal cord injury patient.

But there is still a long way to go to make such centres universal in the NHS. Clearly, we still need to spread the word about CES. Further regular education to healthcare professionals is needed, especially at the primary care level, and that education should come from the patients themselves, as much as the clinical experts.

That is why this book is invaluable not just to CES patients and their doctors, but to the entire population, who need to know what to look out for to enable early diagnosis for themselves and their loved ones and therefore the best chance of recovery.

CLAIRE'S STORY

Jumping from a helicopter and landing on a telegraph pole with a pineapple strapped to the top.

I was thirty-nine when it happened.

I turned over in bed one night in September 2010 and suddenly this pain in my back gripped me, so vice-like I could hardly breathe. It was as if I was instantly paralysed, whilst being electrocuted at the same time. I couldn't move any further. I couldn't get up. It was terrifying. I never cry, but now I burst into tears. My sobs woke my partner Dan, who was sleeping next to me. I had no idea what was happening to me, and he wasn't sure what to do for the best. So, he called 111 and they told me to get to the G.P. in the morning. I didn't exactly need them to tell me that.

The pain was searing. And then I became aware of pins and needles in my buttocks. It felt as if I had enormous weights strapped to each one, as if all the muscle tone had disappeared. It was a sensation I had never felt before. I knew something wasn't right.

In fact, something was very wrong.

I had been having lower back pain and sharp sciatic pain radiating from my hips down my legs for some time, first one leg then the other. The first time I ever had a back problem was about fifteen years before in the mid '90s when my boyfriend at the time assaulted me. He was getting increasingly violent to the point where I was quite used to the odd black eye. But on this occasion, he not only punched me in the eye, but grabbed the hairdryer I'd been using and struck me over the head with it too. That must have sent me to the floor because the next thing I knew I felt him boot me so hard in the lower back I went to jelly. I

5

stayed down until he went out and I knew then I had to get out the flat and not be there when he came back, but when I went to stand up, I could barely walk. So, I crawled out of the flat, across the car park to my car on my hands and knees and managed to drive to my friend's house for safety.

The following day I hobbled to A&E, and they advised bed rest until it got better, which it did after a week or so. From then on, I regularly had a grumbling back, but I thought it was nothing to worry about; it always resolved itself.

In 2003 I started my own cleaning business. Well, I was never very good at being told what to do so it was much better to be my own boss. I employed a few other girls, but did a lot of the cleaning myself, so I could be extra sure the clients got the best service and had nothing to complain about. Shoving a hoover around your own home isn't great on your back but doing it day in day out around other people's homes and offices and hauling equipment in and out of vans over the years, turned that grumbling back pain into sciatica. Being the boss meant nobody told me what to do, but it also meant I didn't feel I could ever take the day off sick, so I told myself to suck it up and get on with it.

However, as time went on, the sciatica became so bad I couldn't stand for long periods or even sleep at night. Queuing in a shop, for example, was impossible and I had to start relying on the girls to do most of the cleaning, while I just supervised; something I was never happy doing. I even started to get strange sensations in my genitals, so I did a bit of googling of my symptoms and that's when Cauda Equina Syndrome popped up: *Cauda Equina Syndrome Medical Emergency.*

(Cauda Equina means horse's tail in Latin and it's the name given to the collection of nerves that splay out from the end of the spinal cord in the shape of a horse's tail. If something compresses these nerves – such as a herniated or bulging disc, a cyst, a tumour or the impact of a car accident – you can feel terrible pain in the lower back and down your legs (sciatica), Your legs may give way, you might experience bladder and bowel dysfunction, pins and needles around your bottom and genitals, or even sexual dysfunction. These symptoms are known as the Red Flags. If these "Red flags" are not acted upon and treatment given quickly enough the result can be permanent disability).

Reading this was unnerving but, with hindsight, a godsend. I had recently been to the G.P. and he had prescribed me some strong painkillers. Two weeks earlier I'd been for an MRI scan at a private hospital on the NHS Choose and Book system, but I hadn't yet had my results. The painkillers made me *feel* slightly better masking the pain, but they didn't deal with the root of the problem. For the next few days, I could move about with more ease, or at least I thought I could, until the night when I turned in bed and a lightning bolt of pain struck me.

My world stopped.

It was 3:30AM and the agony was worse than having a baby – it took my breath completely away. I could only lie there in excruciating pain until the morning. By 8:30 in the morning I was desperate for the loo. I managed to get to the toilet and have a wee. It wasn't only a relief to be able to get myself to the bathroom, but I would later learn how important bladder function is for Cauda Equina Syndrome patients.

Dan had to go off to work, so my eldest daughter, who was eighteen at the time, drove me to the G.P at 10:30AM. I was in such a state, paralysed with pain, it took me quarter of an hour to lower myself into the car.

At the surgery, the doctor's knowledge of back issues was very reassuring and without hesitation he asked me to lie on the examination bed and carried out a sensation test, using his biro to jab around my groin in a 'make do' assessment, as he described it.

'Can you feel that?' he asked.

I shook my head. I was totally numb now around the genitals and the bum (the area that would be in a saddle if you rode a horse, hence the medical name for the lack of sensation in this area: saddle anaesthesia).

'You have Cauda Equina Syndrome,' the doctor said with great authority. 'I'll ring the hospital and get you into the orthopaedic ward straight away.'

I watched through tearful eyes as my G.P. made the call. I overheard the animated conversation as the orthopaedic consultant on the other end of the line refused to see me, fobbing off my G.P, stating I couldn't possibly have Cauda Equina Syndrome (CES) as I was still able to walk. After hanging up, my doctor, clearly furious, wrote a note to the hospital stating that he believed I had Cauda Equina Syndrome. He told me to hand it in at the urgent care centre, stressing that urgent assessment was necessary.

So off I went to the Urgent Care Centre at my local hospital as stipulated by the orthopaedic consultant and whilst waiting to be seen I needed to go to the toilet again. I hobbled off to the loo and went for a wee. But afterwards as I stood up, I noticed there was urine running down my leg, still coming from my bladder, but I couldn't feel it or control it. I mentioned this to the triage nurse, and she wrote it in my notes.

Next, I was assessed by an exhausted looking junior doctor, who was just out of medical school. He was running back and forth between me and the phone to the orthopaedic ward, telling them about the symptoms he was observing, and I was describing, and yet still they refused to accept my G.P's diagnosis of CES.

I was sent home with more painkillers.

I lay on the settee for the rest of the day, feeling the numbness spreading down my legs. At 5PM the G.P. kindly called me to find out how I was. When I explained things were getting worse, he called the hospital and argued with them until they agreed to see me; this time I was told to go to A & E. I wasn't in a hurry to go back there. The thought of moving with this pain was almost too much and they had been no help before, but because my doctor urged me to go and I remembered reading, *Cauda Equina Syndrome Medical Emergency*, I agreed to return. I was terrified of what was happening to my body.

When Dan got home from work, he drove me to the hospital. It was 7:30PM by then and I waited in a cubicle drinking coffee to try and pass the time and distract myself from the pain. After a few cups, I knew I needed a wee but when I went to the loo, I noticed something had changed. It was like trying to pee through a straw. My bladder was full, but only the tiniest stream came out.

Back in the cubicle the pain in my back was so intense everything around me became a blur. I was pleading for help, but I felt ignored and disbelieved.

When I was finally seen, I was subjected to further investigation. The pin prick test was done beneath a blanket, over and over again. The blanket was covered over me so that I couldn't see what the doctor was doing and when. The implication that I was not being truthful about the numbness I was experiencing was hurtful, but not as humiliating as the anal sphincter test – a finger up the bum to test for sensation and the ability to clench – on four different occasions, by four different medical staff.

Four and half hours later, close to midnight, a spinal surgeon came down from a ward and said, as if no one had ever thought of it before, 'I think you could have Cauda Equina Syndrome. You need an MRI scan, let's blue light you over to the spinal surgery centre, shall we?' he smiled.

'Finally, someone is taking this seriously' I thought. Now I would get the treatment I needed, surely.

It was now almost twenty-four hours since we had rung 111. Little did I know then how vital that twenty-four-hour window is for Cauda Equina patients. The clock was ticking, and my window was closing fast.

I was sent for an MRI scan at 3:30AM. I told them I had already had one at a private hospital two weeks before, so they could just contact them to get the results. Apparently, it wasn't that simple. The NHS doctors told me there was no way they could access the information as they didn't share a network with the private hospital.

After having my MRI scan, I wet the bed, my bladder was so full it just overflowed. There was nothing I could do about it. I was so embarrassed. The smell was awful. It turned out I had a raging urine infection because of my bladder dysfunction caused by my creeping CES. I had gone into urinary retention and now my window of opportunity for a full recovery from Cauda Equina Syndrome was firmly shut.

It wasn't any surprise to me when the MRI results came back clearly showing I had a huge herniated L5-S1 disc compressing my cauda equina nerves, slowly killing them off. By the way, the MRI I'd had done at the private hospital weeks earlier had also shown that I had Cauda Equina Syndrome and there was a file on somebody's expensive green leather desktop somewhere stating I needed emergency surgery, but the file had been overlooked and never reported.

At the NHS hospital, they too now stated I needed emergency surgery, but since it was out of hours there was no consultant to do it. The registrar told me that he wanted to do it himself, but the consultant had forbidden him from doing so as it was such a risky procedure. She told him that she would do it first thing in the morning when she arrived at 8AM.

I was confused. If it was an emergency surely it couldn't wait for another five hours? I was also very scared, by now I couldn't feel a thing from my bellybutton down. But I accepted what I was told, along with a much-needed dose of morphine; the pain was all I could think of.

I watched the clock through eyes bloodshot with fatigue and tears and when 8AM came I waited for the consultant to come charging in to save the day. But nobody came.

I eventually went to the operating theatre around midday because *an emergency had come in* that morning, and I was pushed back in the queue.

The surgery, when it did finally happen, involved shaving the herniated part of the disc away, which was compressing my nerves. After a number of hours being compressed these nerves will die, so it is imperative the surgery is done within twenty-four hours of the onset of symptoms such as saddle anaesthesia, bladder issues, and bilateral sciatic leg pain, otherwise the nerves can't bounce back, and you never recover fully. By now, I had been experiencing these acute symptoms for well over thirty-six hours.

Wasn't *that* an emergency?

Since I was completely numb from the waist down before the surgery, the doctors were surprised when, the day after, although I still couldn't feel my legs, I stood up and walked, very tentatively, around. They were I think, expecting me to be in a wheelchair for the rest of my life or a least the foreseeable future.

I had to remain in hospital for a further five days. I was very numb. I couldn't empty my own bowels or bladder. Although I didn't feel it at the time, I can now appreciate how lucky I was to be able to walk around, or rather slowly shuffle, unaided. I was also overjoyed to no longer be feeling any back pain or sciatica. Because of the pain, I hadn't been able to have a decent night's sleep for months so now I slept for a full twenty-four hours, making up for lost time.

More than anything I wanted to get home to my family. The nurses told me I would need to empty my bladder before the hospital could discharge me. So, I went to the toilet several times with a cardboard bowl to perform for the nurses, unaware of what they were really asking. Still, it was difficult to empty my bladder in the normal way. And yet all I could think about was getting out of this hospital. I had a seven-year-old daughter at home. She needed me there. So, I pressed on my stomach, squeezing the urine out of myself so I could report back to the nurses that, yes, I had passed urine, and they let me go. Without asking *how* I passed it or asking if it was normal. I didn't realise at the time that if I was still forcing urine out then I shouldn't have left the hospital. I needed assessment and catheters.

Back home I was so weak and numb in my legs that I resorted to crawling upstairs on my hands and knees. And after seven days of forcing urine from my bladder with unnatural pressures my pelvic floor gave way, my insides were protruding out of my body, I was distraught. I had a uterine prolapse. I called the hospital straight away and left a message explaining what had happened.

No one returned my call.

I called again and again and eventually, four weeks later, I got a call back asking me to come in to get some catheters. However, when I arrived, the nurse who was meant to show me how to use them, had gone early to pick up her child from school and so just left a gift bag of catheters for me to take home. I was handed the bag with no instructions, no demonstration from anyone and left to fend for myself. Yes! it really was a gift bag; it even had a bow. The irony. As many CES patients will tell you cauda equina syndrome is the gift that keeps on giving.

When I got home, I went into the bathroom and with shaking hands poked around trying to find my tiny urethra and then insert a catheter, which is not only frightening but feels humiliating when you first try. You are usually taught how do to this by a urology nurse in hospital. The only way I found I could do it effectively to myself, was standing up so that I had more control over what I was doing. I did it standing over the toilet in case of any accidents and on one of these early occasions Dan walked in and gasped, 'Oh my God! Are you having a pee stood up?' I was devastated. I felt very exposed and vulnerable at the time.

It's a funny story now, but it's humiliating moments like this that pepper your life after CES and can chip away at your morale and sense of dignity. I won't even go into the times I have been incontinent of bowels trying to get upstairs or taking the shortest trip outdoors.

CES patients are often traumatised. They are not taken seriously in the beginning, many are not given the correct assessment or access to MRI scanning and, after surgery, when they need help, there is little or none. CES patients have a reputation for being difficult to deal with – I wonder why? Many have lost trust in the system.

I only found the support I needed via a small Facebook group of around sixty people with Cauda Equina

13

Syndrome, based in the USA. It was through this group that I found out that, as a person with CES, I should be referred into the hospital's urology department for tests on my bladder and that I needed regular trans-anal irrigation for my bowels, which is basically a DIY colonic at home. As far as the uterine prolapse was concerned, I saw a gynaecologist who, after hearing why I was in the state I was, said:

'The way you've been treated is criminal. The only way forward with this is to complain and to get yourself some good legal advice.' The frustration in his voice was something that has always stayed with me.

But that was the last thing on my mind right then. I just wanted to get better and never see the inside of another hospital again.

For most people, things change enormously after CES. It affects all aspects of your life, the professional and the personal. I had to sell my business as I was no longer fit enough to run it, so I found myself financially unstable with a young daughter to look after and another in college. I found walking upstairs impossible and I couldn't feel the floor as my feet were completely numb. I couldn't sit down or stand up for long periods, it was just too painful. I had numerous 'accidents' at home and in public so I had to take a change of clothes wherever I went. One time I decided to touch up the paintwork in the kitchen about a year after my injury and I dropped a heavy tin of paint on my foot. I cut my big toe open and didn't even feel it. I often tripped because I couldn't feel the uneven ground beneath my feet and once, I fell and broke my arm.

My relationship was broken too.

At first Dan was saying all the right things: 'I'll look after you, don't worry.' That was nice to hear, but every night I would cry myself to sleep worrying about my numbness and lack of feeling. For me, this has always been the hardest thing to deal with. Sex had been great before my injury. We'd only been together less than a year, so we were still very much in the honeymoon phase. But now, I had no sexual sensation whatsoever. If I shut my eyes and slept with an entire football team, I would be unaware of it. I was in the prime of my life, not even forty yet. It was devastating. Problems with the bladder and bowels may be one thing, but having my sexuality ripped from me like that played havoc with my sense of identity, my self-esteem.

Dan asked me to marry him – I wondered if it was because he felt sorry for me. I said yes anyway, but our sex life never recovered. I couldn't feel the sensation of his body, which deprived me of that sense of intimacy whilst reinforcing my disability and that, for me, was the most important part of sex. Dan too must have felt disappointed. He tried to have sex with me once or twice, but I knocked him back. I couldn't bear the thought of just lying there feeling nothing. It must have dented his pride too.

The issues I was dealing with were felt huge; the kind of issues those with complete spinal cord injuries deal with, but their injuries are often glaringly obvious by the wheelchairs they use. A lot of people with Cauda Equina Syndrome don't end up in a wheelchair thankfully, but often that means their symptoms and resulting issues are invisible, leaving loved ones and others we deal with, to wonder if we're not just being a bit dramatic.

Consequently, my marriage ended after only eighteen months.

The only people who could relate to what I was going through were the friends I made in the Facebook group, thousands of miles away. They were always available and understood exactly how I felt. I was becoming increasingly aware how little support or information there was for those with Cauda Equina Syndrome. There was no information to be found online about the condition, other than canine CES in dogs. Vets seem to know a lot about it!

Now, sat at home without a job, I felt bereft. I needed to do something to make myself feel useful. And it occurred to me there was something that really needed doing. I decided to set up a my own CES Facebook group where I could share everything I had learnt, signpost others to services and support, and build a strong community. Not only could it be a means of affecting change to try and stop anyone else going through what I and thousands of others had gone through alone, but I also needed to create a new role for myself. My ability to work in a normal job was greatly reduced and I had an overwhelming feeling that this was my purpose in life now. This must be why this had happened to me. A calling if you like.

The NHS admitted liability quite quickly, which you would hope they would do, following the catalogue of errors and delays I've already detailed here. Making a claim for negligence is not an easy thing to do, it's a rollercoaster of emotions and of having to constantly justify yourself and relive what happened to you. The process is long and gruelling and often drawn out for much longer than it should be. After five stressful years I eventually won a settlement from them.

Won.

It's a feeble word to use in this case. I didn't feel like I'd won anything. The money was helpful, necessary even, but I would have given it all back in a heartbeat if I could have my health back again.

When the money arrived, without having to worry about where the next penny was coming from, I was able to invest my time in new skills. I had spent some time volunteering for the Samaritans and for a children's charity. These jobs made me realise that there was not only a need for a support group devoted to CES in England, but that I could be the person to set it up.

I'd always been business minded. Even as a young girl, I used to spend a lot of time with my dad on his fruit and veg stall in Burnley Market. Every Saturday I would watch wide-eyed as he used his patter to sell his produce. I loved this seemingly magic power he had of turning chat into sales. 'Pile it high, sell it cheap,' he used to shout. His drive and passion stuck with me forever.

At home I argued with my Mum a lot. Being rather naïve and thinking I was grown up enough, I decided I was going to move out. I met a guy I thought was amazing and I left. It wasn't my best decision. I never seem to have a good radar when it comes to men. I had gone to an all-girls grammar school, and I put all the problems I had with them later in life down to that. It was with this guy that I had my eldest daughter, who I love dearly and wouldn't swap for the world, but he turned out to be violent. He assaulted me on numerous occasions, including that time when he kicked me in the back, and I went hobbling to A&E. When she was three years old, I couldn't take it anymore. I finally found the courage to leave him and checked us into a domestic violence unit.

So, there I was in my mid-twenties on my own with a young daughter. I had no one to support me financially and recalling my love of the busy market at Burnley, I got a stall at Blackburn where I would sell clothes for nights out. Later, I got a job as an account manager for a mobile phone company. I loved meeting purchase managers and forming relationships with them and as I rose through the ranks, it spurred me on to think about business development.

17

A few years on and I met the man who became the father of my second daughter. She was born in 2002. But her dad turned out to be as much use as a chocolate teapot. He was never keen on contributing so I was the main bread winner, which meant I quickly went back to work after having our baby and he would look after her in the daytime. He couldn't cope with that, so I had to give up my job and find something that worked around looking after the baby too. The only way I could really do this, I thought, was to start my own cleaning business. I went from being a senior sales executive in charge of corporate accounts to cleaning toilets. But at least it was my own business, and I was determined to make it a successful one.

It did well. I made good money, and I could look after my family myself. It wasn't exactly a glamourous job, but I felt empowered by it. Me and the girls worked hard, and we had a good time after hours too. I loved going out with my friends.

When I drove my daughter to nursery before work we would sing along to songs in the van. *One Love* by the boyband Blue was one of our favourites and she knew the words inside out. Little did I know how Blue and I, would become inextricably linked by CES in the future.

Right then life was good. However, the work soon became very intensive, my drive to make a success of anything I did, had me working myself into the ground. After about seven years of pushing myself in this way my back got worse and then came the fateful night when my CES manifested, and everything changed.

So that's when I began devoting all my time to setting up an organisation that could help others with CES and perhaps stop it happening so frequently in the future. I knew if I could utilise that hungry businesswoman in me and pour those skills into this new venture, I could generate funds and resources for the charity in a very significant way. It didn't really feel like a choice to me. It felt like I had to do it and would always need to do it until things changed.

By *sorted* I mean a complete systemic change. A seamless pathway from G.P, A&E, surgery and through to rehab as opposed to the obstacles and issues that exist now. If I get my way, everyone with back pain will be triaged and safety netted for Cauda Equina Syndrome. It's such a time sensitive issue that it must surely be better to think in these preventative ways, since a cure is often off the table if it's left too late. We need more MRI slots to confirm the diagnosis and more radiographers who can read them. More training for healthcare professionals and patients, as well as more resources for the NHS. We also need to change the societal attitude that those who complain of back pain are just skivers looking for a few weeks off work. Glass back syndrome, I like to call it.

One woman, who our organization is helping right now, discovered that on her notes from A & E, the nurse had simply scrawled, *trying to get more drugs*. A different attitude would have saved our friend a lifetime of pain and suffering.

I needed funds, so I applied for a couple of grants at first, one being a social enterprise grant, which I was awarded to set up a website. I then created a LinkedIn account and started to connect with anybody and everybody who might have an interest in Cauda Equina Syndrome. I used my connections to generate income for the website and marketing. I approached medical professionals who offered their support and found that there were a few trying to change things for cauda equina patients.

There were, I soon discovered, many types of firms that would be happy to be associated with a charity like the one I wanted to set up and I began to ring around. I only contacted the best of the best: the best medical device suppliers, the best legal advisors, the best medical experts. Integrity is at the core of what we do. I wanted to put the patient first and to give them a collective voice. Our new corporate partnerships added to the coffers considerably, turning my social enterprise into a fully-fledged charity. With that money added to other fundraising, we could provide services for people with CES that just didn't exist then, such as psychosexual counselling, guided meditation for pain management, a buddy mentoring service, support group meetings, training for medical professionals, to name but a few.

As the founder of the Cauda Equina Champions Charity, I found myself invited to various Cauda Equina events and attended one in a leading rehabilitation centre. The first speaker was an orthopaedic surgeon, who began his address, incredibly, with this:

'People presenting with back pain at A&E are from the periphery of society and are merely clogging up the system.'

There is so much prejudice around back pain.

Of course, there are those who lay it on thick to get a few weeks off work, but it only takes a few more minutes of assessment to work out if there are Red flags pointing to Cauda Equina Syndrome; a few minutes well spent for both the patient's health and the NHS if they don't want to waste any more cash on negligence settlements.

From 2015 – 2020 there were 535 claims made from CES patients who had been let down by the system and it cost the NHS £437,000,000. That's about £87,000,000 a year. It takes less than £87,000,000 per year to run the eleven specialist spinal units in England. If we could eliminate claims made through negligence to CES sufferers, the NHS could double the number of spinal units in the country. It's an incredible thought.

I married again shortly after my settlement to an old boyfriend I used to know when I went out with the girls in the cleaning company. After the disaster of my first marriage, which was due in part to my insecurity around my sexual dysfunction since CES, I kept my sexual issues a secret from this new partner; after all, he knew the old me, the person I still wanted to be. I am not proud of that, but this is how CES can mess with your self-esteem and mental health. I was still trying to work out who this new me was and I was unsure of how he would react if he knew. Although I believed I was in love with him, I never fully trusted him, and I had a feeling he would use my lack of sexual function and continence issues against me if he knew. It turns out I was right to mistrust him. I eventually realised he only wanted to marry me after he found out about the money I had got from the settlement with the NHS.

I managed to get a divorce after a lot of bullying from him, but it really highlights the issues that CES can throw up. The fact that so much of the condition is invisible to the outside world is the root of so many of these issues: from surgeons not appreciating the syndrome because you're managing to walk around, to sexual dysfunction, bladder and bowel issues, chronic pain, and the way it impacts your mental health, to the stigma around seeking compensation for avoidable trauma and injuries; devastating life changing injuries

In my work with the Cauda Equina Champions Charity, I find myself in meetings with people from companies that supply devices to help with sexual issues for spinal injury patients. They tell me about vacuum pumps for the penis, ejaculation stimulators, penile implants, all manner of things, in case Viagra doesn't work for you.

'And what do you have for women?' I ask.

'Well...' they routinely stutter, 'Um...'

Since the dawn of time, women's sexuality has always been ignored by the patriarchal society we live in. And now our sexual dysfunction is equally neglected. And this becomes more of a problem when you realise that over half of CES sufferers are women. This is due in part to the kind of professions women tend to undertake and childbirth I imagine. A lot of carers and nurses, with all the lifting and bending they have to do, suffer with CES, and the majority of them are women. The condition used to be a problem for the older generations, for those older than forty, but nowadays there are many more young women in particular presenting with CES after pushing themselves too far in the gym to achieve that Instagrammable body.

Ten years on from my injury, my muscle tone has improved and sensation in my feet returned a little. I can't say when it happened, but one day I trod on a sharp stone and was dumbfounded, ecstatic even, that I could feel it. I have more awareness of the ground beneath me now, so I don't trip or fall as often. I don't have to use catheters anymore to empty my bladder, but my bowels never improved. I have no feeling there to know when I need to go, so I still irrigate regularly. But at least I know how to do it and have the device to help. It's empowering to be able to do this for myself and not rely on medical staff. Some people are not told these devices exist, so they become housebound, unable to go out for fear of being incontinent. Ten percent of Cauda Equina patients go on to have a stoma bag fitted because their bowels don't work at all.

On the downside for me, the pain in the buttocks and rectum has never gone away. The best way I can describe it is that I feel as if I've been dropped by a helicopter from a great height onto a telegraph pole with a pineapple strapped to the top of it. It makes for some bizarre dreams at night, I can tell you. I live with that feeling of having been rammed up the arse with a spiky fruit-topped mast 24/7 and it's exhausting.

It took me most of those ten years to really come to terms with who I am now. The trainwreck of my second divorce made me take a good look at myself and started me on the long road to rehabilitation, mentally speaking as well as physically. The adjustment people with CES have to make is massive and there's still a lack of mental health support for them. Our condition and our issues may often be invisible, but *we* should not be – something we at the Cauda Equina Champions Charity are trying to redress.

There are many dedicated medical professionals working very hard now to improve things for Cauda Equina Syndrome patients; an undertaking undoubtedly driven by the increasing amount of clinical negligence cases and compensation payments. These figures are sadly set to increase further before we see real improvement across the county. But it is coming.

I owe a debt of gratitude to my own G.P, Dr White. If he hadn't taken the time to ring me at the end of his working day, to see how I was after being rebuffed at A&E, I have no doubt in my mind I would be in a wheelchair right now. My pain would be something I would not be able to tolerate without huge doses of morphine and medication. I know this because I have met others far worse off than me who nobody fought for. I would have stayed on my settee waiting for my pain to go, and not gone back to hospital that day. My life would be so much harder. Thank you, Dr White, I am eternally grateful.

MARTIN'S STORY

The Comeback King

Christmas holds some weird connotations for me these days. Horrible events always seem to happen then. The most significant of which was December 23, 2017.

It was a Saturday, and I was rushing around because I was on my way to do my Christmas shopping. I was never one for planning ahead as far as that was concerned. Even though I had loads to do, I nipped into the gym on my way to the shops. Training was very important to me. I would always make time for that. During the session, I was dead lifting (lifting a bar stacked with weights from the floor until you're standing up straight with the bar at your hips) when my left foot slipped halfway through the lift. The next thing I knew I was on my back.

And I couldn't feel my legs.

Was it carelessness on my part? Was it just a freak accident? Was my mind on getting round the packed shops before they closed, instead of focusing on the technique I needed to do the lift? Who knows really? What I do know, is that nothing was ever the same again.

Nearly ten years before in 2004, I was in my mid-twenties and working in sales and marketing. I had studied Management at university in Lancashire where I'd grown up, and then Business Management as a Master's degree, but I wasn't happy in my work. I had this feeling that everything I'd done in life I'd done to make other people happy or fulfil their expectations of me. My father was a senior partner in a reputable accounting firm and had a very conventional view on what you should do for a living. So, I had gone down that path for a while, but now I was sure that it was time to do something for me.

I'd been going to the gym since I was sixteen years old and enjoyed weight training. Fitness had become a passion of mine and so I decided to get the relevant qualifications and started a new career as a personal trainer.

At the gym one day, I met someone who competed in the sport of powerlifting. He had seen me training and said, 'Martin, you'd be great as a powerlifter. Have you ever thought about doing it competitively?'

The idea of attempting to win a competition really appealed to me. I was never one for football, rugby, and the other sports my mates did, but the thought of getting some trophy or whatever, for lifting would really add to that sense of personal achievement I was looking for when I started my new career in fitness.

I went to see a few competitions at first, just to get a feel for what I was letting myself in for. The idea of getting up on stage in front of everyone and showing what I could do was a bit daunting, but also very exciting. I was quickly hooked and a year later in 2008 I entered my first competition. It was a qualifier for the British Championships. I had no designs on the championship itself, but it would be a bit of a dream come true to at least qualify for it.

It was a small event in a sports hall, but there was a decent sized audience and three judges scrutinizing the nine lifts I had to do and so the adrenaline rush was like nothing I'd felt before. I also met lots of great people in the powerlifting community who quickly became firm friends.

Despite the low expectations I had of myself, I did qualify for the British finals and suddenly found myself there at the Bournemouth International Centre with TV cameras trained on me as the event was broadcast on Sky

Sports. It was a total buzz and I ended up coming fifth, so to say I was pleased with that is a serious understatement. I felt like a bit of rockstar as the crowds cheered; it was addictive. The following year in 2009 I was back at the qualifiers. I had worked hard that year, improved a lot and learned a bit about the tactics of competition so I decided to lift in the next weight category down from the one I had been in the previous year, which meant I didn't have to compete against these monsters who were much bigger than me. Bulk is everything in powerlifting, so being near the top of the 100-kilo category was more advantageous for me, though I did often just scrape in at 99.9 kilos.

I was gob-smacked, as were many of the community who had never heard of this new kid on the block – when I qualified and then won my weight class at the British Championships.

By now I even had sponsorship from Myprotein, who had seen the training log I had kept on their forum (we're still in the days before social media was a thing). They thought my approach and drive was a good fit for their image. I found myself doing photo shoots and exhibitions alongside famous fitness celebrities like Ross Edgley, and I was loving it. It's not like I could give up the day job, but I had all the protein shakes I could handle and was training a couple of hours four days a week incorporating a lot of work on core strength and technique – lifting badly is not an option with such heavy weights.

In 2009 I qualified for the British team at the World Championships, where I came second in my weight class; second only to one of the greatest powerlifters there has ever been, so I was more than happy with that.

In 2010, as I approached my thirtieth birthday, I won my weight class and won the overall title of *best male lifter* in the British finals. Now everything in my life was revolving around powerlifting. Planning for the next competition and working towards it got me out of bed in the morning. I would shuffle my work as a personal trainer around so I could prioritize my own training and take days off here and there to attend competitions. Luckily my partner, who I'd been with since 2003, would come with me to competitions and was supportive… For now.

I was invited to the World Championships in Argentina that year and was gutted not to be able to attend because of some niggling injuries. It made me understand that I wasn't totally indestructible anymore, now I was in my thirties. This was brought home to me even more powerfully when the following year, I was demonstrating an exercise to a client at work and twisted my knee, tearing the cartilage from the bones above and below the joint. I needed surgery to remove some of the cartilage and fix some of the other damage. Even though I could barely walk on that leg for a while I couldn't let go of powerlifting, so decided to enter a couple of bench press competitions (which involves lying down to push the weights from your chest, so no standing needed). My partner now thought I was a bit bonkers.

'When are you going to give it up?' she'd say.

'When something stops me,' was my flippant response.

To me that thing would probably be age, but as far as my partner was concerned, the thing that would stop me would be marriage and kids.

We did get married in 2013 and shortly after that, with the help of a physio at my workplace, I was able to do focus on my knee and get myself fit enough to start lifting again. I thought I'd take it easy at first and do a little test run at a small competition at a gym in London, but it turned into me breaking the British squat record on two of my three lifts.

I was back.

But this time, my wife was not as supportive. She had thought that we would settle down and have kids soon after getting married. I had taken a management position at the fitness club I had been a personal trainer in, so I had a much more secure and regular income conducive to starting a family, but powerlifting quickly dominated my life again. I was quite a shy, introverted kind of bloke before I discovered lifting, but now I was bursting with confidence. I felt so good about myself I didn't want to think about anything else but the sport that was giving me this buzz.

As the cracks began to show in my relationship, I found myself whizzing off to the Czech Republic for the European Championships, winning my weight class, breaking the *three lift* record, and generally having a fantastic time for a week in beautiful Prague. It was summer, the weather was amazing, I was with all my teammates and, although the day before the weigh-in we were all just drinking water and avoiding eating, after competition day we hit the bars and the restaurants and gorged on beer and food in celebration of a job well done.

Back home, my relationship was beyond repair. I had more than a feeling that my wife had been getting the attention she wasn't getting from me from another bloke, and so on Christmas Eve I walked out. There's such a pressure for families to come together at Christmas and for everything to be picture perfect that it forces a lot of people to see how broken and anything-but-perfect their families are.

So, it was Christmas, I was thirty-four and I was sleeping on the floorboards in my mum's loft because she only had a one bedroomed bungalow. It sounds like a bit of a sad situation, but I will admit I was happy, even relieved.

And I had powerlifting. What more could I need?

The following year I was invited to do a professional competition in Ireland where I won a bit of money and drank a lot of Guinness and by 2016, I was the overall winner at the European Championships. I was still breaking records and so I went into the next competition with a headstrong attitude that I was going to push myself to even greater heights, or rather weights.

On the first lift of that competition, as I squatted down, the quad muscle in my leg tore. That was me, out of the competition and out of training, perhaps for good. That sent me into a bit of a downward spiral mentally and I had to take a month off work with depression. Lifting meant so much to me, looking forward to the next competition was everything, and now without it, I didn't know what to do with myself.

Luckily, I could do a lot of rehabilitation on my leg with the experts at my workplace and by 2017 I was back competing internationally. This took me to places I'd never been, winning gold medals at a world class level for the first time.

Things were great again, and they were even greater when, in November of that year, I got together with a work colleague I had known for some time. Zoe was a stunner. We got on famously and, because she had been through a divorce like me, we had a lot of the same attitudes to life and relationships.

Then Christmas came.

That day when I'd nipped into the gym to do a bit of training before cramming in the shopping. And I found myself flat on my back, my legs going numb.

I was convinced I had torn my hamstring muscles in both legs, hence my inability to move them. My colleagues rushed over and took the weights away, offering to call an ambulance, but I reckoned I'd be OK after a while. I wasn't in any great pain, just numb, so they helped me roll onto my front where I rested for a bit, expecting to be able to get up soon enough. Instead, I soon felt this intense pins and needles in my legs, the kind you get if you've slept on your arm for hours, and severe pain. However, with this feeling, as horrible as it was, came a bit of movement in my legs, so with the help of my colleagues, I staggered out to my car and, perhaps foolishly in hindsight, I managed to drive home to Zoe's flat.

By the time I got there, the pain and intense pins and needles had got so bad Zoe called 111. They asked various questions to try and assess my situation. The pain was much greater when I tried to stand up and the tingling and numbness was now everywhere from the waist down. So, the operator called an ambulance.

Two hours later, the pain was much worse, and the ambulance still hadn't arrived, so Zoe cancelled it, got me into the car and drove me to Bolton A&E.

When I arrived, a nurse gave me some painkillers while we waited to see a doctor. When he eventually came, he seemed distracted, rushing around, which was understandable as the place was heaving with Christmas accidents. Once we had his attention, he seemed very focused on my back and quite dismissive of the strange sensations I was having in my legs, groin, and genitals. He said he was going to refer me, and I'd have to wait for a letter in the post.

'Do you know when it will be?' I asked.

He shrugged. 'Might be a few weeks.'

A few weeks? I could tell something was seriously wrong with me and so I was sure a few weeks was not good enough. I had a BUPA healthcare plan, so I asked the doctor to write a letter to them instead so I could get a scan. He obliged, but when we got home that night and rang BUPA we found out they were closed for four days over Christmas. Bloody Christmas!

Now my symptoms were getting more complex. I was struggling to go to the toilet. I was drinking plenty but nothing much was coming out. I spent Christmas Day lying on the bed and insisted Zoe went off to see her family, so at least one of us could have a good time.

That night I spent in agony, sinking my teeth into the pillow as the painkillers stopped doing their job. There wasn't a position I could get myself into where I didn't feel excruciating pain, so Zoe took me back to A&E on Boxing Day and we intended not to leave until we got some answers.

A different doctor this time took us very seriously. In fact, she seemed to be panicking after she carried out a pin prick test, knowing that something needed to be done quickly, but not knowing quite what it was. I was catheterised to help me empty my bladder, which was by this time swollen, while the doctor called another hospital for advice. When she came back to us, she told me I needed an MRI as a matter of urgency and an ambulance with blue lights flashing would be taking me to the hospital in Salford where they had the resources to do it.

Six hours later the ambulance arrived.

After a couple of hours of waiting in a wheelchair for it, I'd been found a bed, and after a couple of hours of being in the bed, Zoe was telling the doctors she could just drive me to Salford, no need to keep waiting for the ambulance. The trouble was the hospital said it couldn't let

Zoe drive us as we were now under the care of the hospital and transporting me to Salford was their responsibility.

We got to Salford at 11PM and I had the scan around midnight. A few hours later a doctor showed me the images from the MRI explaining that he thought part of one of the discs in my back had moved into the spinal canal, but he needed to discuss it further with other colleagues to form a plan of action. They kept me in the hospital that night in a spinal injury unit and when the doctor returned, he told me surgery was necessary to stop the pressure being exerted on the nerves. He also said that although the surgery would stop things getting worse, there was no guarantee it could fix the damage already done.

The consultant went through the disclaimer form that I had to sign. Of course, these things are necessary to explain all risks, however small, and not to give false hope, but I was told there was a risk I could be incontinent, a risk I could never walk again, even a small risk that, because of being such a big bloke and the 'all fours' position I would have to be in to have the surgery done that the anaesthesia could ruin my eyesight. This was so overwhelming that my only reaction was to laugh and say to the anaesthetist, 'Well, if I can't walk ever again, and I'm blind, do me a favour and just don't wake me up.'

Zoe wasn't laughing, but the consultant reassured me that having the operation was my only chance of getting any better, so I signed the form.

When I came round, I was told the surgery had been a success. The intensity of the burning pain I had in my back and legs before the operation, had definitely subsided. But I still couldn't walk on my own, which was frightening. I had to be taken for a shower by a nurse and then lay in bed on my back for a few days, having regular scans of my

33

bladder which seemed to show that I was still retaining urine. Then a doctor came and told me that they weren't sure the scanner was working properly, so I might not be retaining as much urine as they first thought. I was reassured that I would see the surgeon again in about six weeks to check on my progress and meanwhile, if I wanted to go home, I could.

Zoe took me home. It was painful and very difficult trying to get into the car but at least I had my considerable upper body strength to help pull myself in and out and then hang onto a walking frame Zoe had bought to help me get into the flat.

I spent weeks laying on the bed, bored out my brains, on a lot of painkillers and still not able to go to the toilet properly. In bed at night, I would often have accidents with my bladder or bowels and needed Zoe's help to get cleaned up. I had gone from a confident strong sixteen stone bloke with a sixpack who felt on top of the world – and indeed was top in the world in his chosen sport – to needing my girlfriend to change me and the bed, because I couldn't control myself. I felt humiliated, as if I'd lost all dignity, and Zoe, though she was an absolute angel, must have thought, just a couple of months into our relationship, 'This is not what I signed up for.'

We had spent our time together planning weekends away, being romantic, everything was quite literally roses, but now I found myself disabled and Zoe had become my carer. I would cry in the middle of the night as I wet the bed yet again and there was no way I could stop it, no way I could take the pressure off Zoe. I felt like a burden to her. I felt useless.

I had no feeling in my genitals sexually speaking and that was such a blow to my self-esteem that, believe it or not, I would have traded never being able to walk again for a functioning sex life. I had a wheelchair that I could use to still get around while my legs were not working, but there was nothing that could replace the loss of function in what I thought at the time, made me a man.

And then finally the day came to see the surgeon again.

When we arrived at his office on a Monday late afternoon, he had his winter coat on as if he was ready to go. He asked me if the pain was better, which I could tell him it was, but I was still very sore.

'Well, it can take eighteen months to recover from such a significant injury,' he chirped. 'Now let's have a look at your scar!'

I showed him my back. He seemed very happy with his work and then tried to send us on our way.

At this Zoe became very agitated. 'But he can't walk or go to the toilet properly. What can we do about that?'

'See your G.P.' he said.

And that was that.

We were both deeply frustrated. Perhaps we'd expected more from the surgeon than was in his remit, but we had no idea what the future would hold for us and what help we might need or get.

I had a copy of my discharge notes from the hospital and that was the first time throughout this entire nightmare that I became aware of the words *Cauda Equina Syndrome*. In the haze of those first hours in Salford, I think I'd read them on the disclaimer form, but I had never been told what they meant. So, I started googling and that's when I came across the Cauda Equina Champions Charity and Claire.

She was brilliant and told me exactly which departments I should be getting referrals to, so armed with this knowledge I did go back to my G.P. and he referred me to a neurologist, who was a fantastic help. He made some assessments and then referred me to the continence team, got me on some good pain medication and put everything in perspective for me. Finally, a couple of months after the surgery I felt as if my recovery was really beginning.

I bought a lightweight wheelchair which I could get myself in and out of and chuck in the car myself, so I could start to get around without Zoe's help. It was an ex-demonstration one, so I managed to get it for half price, but still it set me back a thousand pounds, which was a shock – I had no idea how much stuff like that cost. Nevertheless, it was priceless for my sense of independence. Luckily, my feet worked well enough to control the pedals in the car, but my knees and hips just wouldn't allow me to balance and hold myself up, in order to walk. Thankfully, all that work I'd done on my upper body as a powerlifter came in handy when I needed to haul myself about.

I was able to go back to work where I could use the swimming pool and the generous services of the physio there to work on my balance. I felt so blessed to have the resources there at my workplace that some people with my condition would struggle to find. I started to feel quite positive again. I saw the rehab as a challenge, a bit like training for a competition, and every time I made some improvement in my legs I felt like a champion. I gained a little more control in my bladder and bowels, but after about six months the progress seemed to plateau, and it dawned on me that I would never be completely fine again.

This had a huge impact on my mental health. I sank into a depression and although Zoe never complained about looking after me where I needed it, I found it hard to accept that Zoe was happy staying with me. She was a good-looking, outgoing person, surely, she'd rather be with someone else. In my dark times I kept trying to press her buttons to find out, and we'd argue. After one particularly blazing row, I got in the car and left. I went to my mum's that night and took a razor blade to my legs to numb the physical and the mental pain. I took a handful of sleeping pills but luckily, I woke up the next morning. That was when I knew it was time to get some counselling.

The counselling helped me comprehend that depression is a completely normal reaction in someone who has gone through what I went through. I didn't have to feel weak because I wasn't coping. It was absolutely, par for the course. It would be weird not to feel down after such a life-changing experience.

This helped me build bridges with Zoe and in 2019 we bought a bungalow together. Not only was this a practical help for me with everything on one floor but also the fact that we did it together filled me with a sense of security as we both committed to this next step in life side by side.

Over the next year or so I began to recover a little more. I started using a stick or the frame to walk around the house and I got the necessary device so I could irrigate my own bowels regularly. It's not the most pleasant thing in the world to do, it's time consuming and rather painful, but it gives you reassurance that you're not going to have frequent bowel accidents, which is far more important, and gets rid of the awful feeling of having a football eternally stuck up your arse.

Nowadays, my bladder is almost under control through daily self-catheterisation and timing toilet visits regularly, as I don't sense when my bladder is full, although I do still have some episodes of leaking. My balance is bad. I have hardly any sensation in my legs, but I can walk short distances unaided if I concentrate. I rely on a walking stick or a crutch when I go out and about as my legs are wobbly, and I continue to need my wheelchair for any longer journeys, days out and holidays.

I have spent a huge amount of time working on regaining some muscle tone. My obsession with training before the injury definitely helped me have the stamina to carry on working on my recovery in those extremely dark times. And this is essential. I began attending groups run by the CES charity and when I listened to other people's stories, I understood that sometimes the biggest barrier to recovery was lacking the drive to push on through the pain, which you have to have if you're going to get stronger. Obviously, I had a physical advantage and the right mindset already to do this for myself, but this world champion also had further to fall. The toll on my mental health was huge, and in many respects will continue to be a lifelong battle. I've been extremely close to suicide, had bouts of self-harm, and spent many nights hoping to never wake up. I will never powerlift again, but if my powerlifter's drive can inspire other people with CES to push on through their own obstacles and improve their quality of life, even slightly, then my injury has not been completely in vain.

These days I try to find pleasure in other things that don't involve physical prowess, such as painting and drawing. I'm learning that it's OK to be rubbish at things – at least at first – and I am beginning to enjoy the journey of improving in my creative pursuits, just as I enjoyed improving in the early days of lifting, until enjoyment was replaced with an obsession with results. Now my output doesn't have to impress anyone else – no audience, no judges – just me.

I realized that by obsessing over powerlifting, it stopped being as much fun, and actually the most pleasure I got in life was helping others improve in my role as a personal trainer. That is why I'd like to spend time now helping other people who live with CES and promoting mental health awareness, especially to other men, because men are generally rubbish at asking for help. Our masculine pride gets in the way, and that is why three times more men commit suicide than women. When people look at me, they often see an alpha male type and, in many ways, I fitted that stereotype before my injury. But when I lost my sexual function particularly, it really challenged my perception of what it was to be a man. When I hit rock bottom, I knew I had to stop trying to solve every problem myself (a typical masculine trait) and start sharing my problems, something women are generally much better at doing. So, I'd like to inspire other people now to do the same. A great man, I'm learning, is someone who lifts other people up emotionally, and not just someone who can lift enormous weights.

I would like to express my wholehearted thanks to both Dr Shakespeare of the NHS and Claire Thornber from the Cauda Equina Champions Charity, without whom I would never have known about the support or specialist services available post CES or have had any access to them, to help improve my quality of life. The rehabilitation through these services has enabled me to manage my condition better day to day and continue trying to live my life. Thank you.

JAMES'S STORY

Little Wins and Smashing Goals

We were all about making memories.

No matter how busy we were, no matter how hectic our work schedules, Kate and I were determined to take our kids away on at least one holiday abroad every year and weekends away wherever possible. We all loved camping, so we explored everything the British Isles had to offer when we weren't going abroad. Cornwall was a favourite destination. We wanted the kids to look back at their childhoods with all the joy that we looked back at ours. Our own families were important to us and now Kate and I were building a new picture-perfect family together.

We had married in 2016 in our late twenties and now in 2020, we lived in the idyllic New Forest near the south coast of England with our two gorgeous kids, Lily, who was five, and Freddie who was only eighteen months old.

But it had been no walk in the park to get to this stage.

Six months before we married my dad died of dementia. It really knocked me off balance. Not just because dementia is such a harrowing way to go, but because I couldn't believe I was losing a parent when I was still in my twenties. That's not how things are supposed to go, are they?

My dad had me later in life, so he was not exactly a spring chicken when he became ill. He was a bit of a hero to me. I loved his optimism, his cockney Blitz Spirit, cultivated by growing up along the Old Kent Road in southeast London. He was not one to cry over spilt milk, always had a smile on his face, always saw the bright side and was devoted to his family. I was proud when people saw those same traits in me. I loved being a chip off the old block.

But when Dad got dementia, this little chip had to grow up too fast. Suddenly I felt all manner of alien pressures. I was arranging power of attorney documents and my sister, who was already a care assistant in a residential home, was trying to look after Dad at her house. She made such a valiant effort, but since she had three young children and an exhausting job in care already, this was not sustainable, and we soon had to move dad into a care home.

We felt so bad about putting him in a home, but we made sure that it was right on the beachfront in Bournemouth, because it had always been his dream to have a view of the sea. We would take him down to the promenade in his wheelchair to the spots he used to take us to as children, when he was making memories for us.

It was so tough to see him losing those memories. He would often say when we visited, 'The staff tell me you're my children. But how do I know this is true?'

It was hard to see my sister washing and cleaning him and putting him in incontinence pads just as he and Mum used to do to us when we were babies. It was sad to have to sell his home and watch the proceeds disappear to pay the whopping care bill for the eighteen months he'd spend in that facility. It wasn't right.

When the inevitable happened and Dad died, my big sister took it badly. She had devoted so much time and energy to looking after him and yet still, even with all her expertise, she couldn't combat this awful condition. She crumbled and I realised I would have to step up and deal with all the administrative stuff that comes with death, when it is the last thing, you feel like dealing with. I was working my way up at a high street bank at the time, so at least all the financial nuts and bolts that needed sorting were already in my ballpark. But when everything was done and dusted, about six months after Dad died, I realised I had been on autopilot the whole time. I suddenly came up for air and that was when the grief hit me.

Now I crumbled too.

I was not only grieving the loss of my hero but grieving the loss of the last couple of years during which I spent every day at the care home and therefore neglected my wife and Lily, who was barely a year old at the time. The guilt coupled with the loss sent me into a deep bought of depression. My employers at the bank were very sympathetic. They gave me time off where I needed it and a phased return to work while I sought counselling to help me get back on track. When I did go back to work full time, I thought of how my dad was so proud of me working in a bank and how he would always encourage me to push myself in life. I could sometimes be a bit reticent about that, not quite believing I was good enough to be anyone's boss, but now, realising how short life is, I knew I had nothing to lose, so I began to pour all my efforts into climbing the ranks at work, to continue to make my dad proud. And before I knew it, I had gone from an advisor to the manager of the branch.

Kate was very supportive as she was very career driven too. She was a senior cardiac physiologist in the local hospital. Her shifts were brutal, she was regularly on call at the weekends and her job meant she had to deal with death frequently, so she'd had to develop the skill of switching off from work when the working day was done. I, however, was so over the moon that I had clinched a job as a manager at my age, that I would struggle to switch off when I got home – I didn't want to do anything to jeopardize my position at the bank. I carried on pushing myself for the next promotion to senior manager, in charge of several banks, not just meeting all my development targets, but smashing them.

Then in 2019 Kate was pregnant again.

Kate had endured a miscarriage after Lily and so when she got pregnant with Freddie, we were treading on eggshells the whole time fearing the worst. When it was time to give birth, the labour was long and traumatic for both Kate and Freddie. He emerged into the world a ghostly shade of blue and so he was immediately whisked away from Kate for lifesaving treatment. Kate could not see her new-born son and was desperately asking me what was going on and how he was. I could see the doctors working on him, trying to resuscitate his lifeless body, and I knew Kate needed reassurance more than anything right then, just as I did when I was losing my dad. She didn't need to see me freaking out, so I told her he was going to be OK and luckily, after a long time in intensive care, he was.

However, when we finally got Freddie home, Kate felt something wasn't right. She could not feel that natural maternal connection you expect to feel, that she had had with Lily when she was born. Even as our new baby son cried, Kate would look at Freddie emotionlessly. It was so upsetting to witness. She knew she needed help and so we sought counselling, during which she discovered that she was suffering from PTSD, a result of the difficulties in labour and being separated from Freddie immediately after he was born. The counselling was very sensitively handled and therefore very effective. I was so proud of the way Kate came through this and happy we could get through it together as a team.

Now working hard to fund those holidays and make those memories was more vital than ever.

Keeping fit was important too. I liked running and in the New Forest there was no shortage of beautiful places to train. I enjoyed setting myself goals, just like I did at work, pushing myself further and further each time: little wins that added up to one big triumph.

And then COVID-19 made the world stop.

Kate, working in the NHS, didn't stop at all: she found herself working even more hours than she did before. And, although I was working from home for a while, running a bank from your living room is just not feasible. There was great pressure on me to return to the branch, but with Kate working so much, I was also needed at home to look after the kids.

During lockdown, as most people discovered, going out for some exercise was one of those few times you could get out of the house and feel a little sense of freedom. Since running was my exercise and the vast New Forest gave you all the social distancing you could wish for, I made the most of it, but by the end of summer 2020 my legs weren't happy. I had pains radiating down the back of my legs, but I didn't want to give up running, so I thought I'd just tape my legs up like serious runners do when necessary. Before long, my legs were mummified in tape, and I smelt like an Asian Spa as I applied all manner of heat rubs and tiger balms into what I assumed were just aching muscles. Then, came that fateful week I can never forget.

SUNDAY

We had arranged with friends to go out on a walk in the forest while the summer weather was still holding up, but when they arrived at our house raring to go, I told them

'I'm so sorry guys, I'm going to have to give it a miss. My legs are just killing me.'

My friends joked around as we always did. 'Don't be a pussy! Man up! It's just a stroll in the woods, not a marathon.'

I laughed and any other day that might have been enough to get me out, but this time I knew I needed to stay put. I couldn't explain what it was, but I knew it was more than aching legs, so I made my apologies and everyone else went out for the walk without me.

When Kate got back, she said, 'How are you doing?'

'I don't know,' I replied, 'but I don't think this is just muscular pain.'

MONDAY

We needed to do the weekly shop. We took the kids and went around stocking up on essentials and despairing at the shelves devoid of toilet rolls. Then when we came through the checkout Freddie, as toddlers do, made an unsteady run for the automatic door. I instinctively ran after him and scooped him up in my arms before he ended up under the wheels of a car and then…

POP!!!

I'm not sure if this was a sound that my body really made, but it was how it felt. As if something inside me had burst or snapped. And now I could hardly move.

'You alright?' Kate said.

'Not really,' I said, but we had kids and shopping to get home so we – well, Kate, while I winced and hobbled – got the little ones and the bags into the car. But getting myself in was almost impossible. I couldn't just bend and sit in the usual way. When I twisted to put my legs into the car the pain was how I imagine being electrocuted might feel, or how I would respond if a red-hot poker was plunged through my flesh. I had to fold myself, hugging my knees towards my chest to stand any chance of getting into a seated position and yet all the while, I felt shards of glass dragging along my back.

There was no doubt something was very wrong.

I was so glad when we got home and I could just lay down and rest up until this, whatever it was, passed. But there wasn't a position I could get into that didn't feel like bolts of electricity firing through my back and legs. It was unbearably painful, until I discovered that being on my front on the floor splayed out like a starfish, with a pillow under my chin took the edge off the spasms. And I watched TV with my kids from this bizarre angle to distract myself from the pain. If I had to move around I could only do so on my hands and knees to avoid the spasms kicking back in. I knew I had a high tolerance for pain, but this just brought me to tears.

Kate offered to help me up to bed as it got late.

'No, no, I'm fine,' I said like a typical bloke. 'I'll sort it. I'll be up in a bit.'

But I wasn't up in a bit. I couldn't stand up anymore. And eventually, after trying in vain to drag myself along the sofa, I called my wife on her mobile because I didn't even have the breath to shout upstairs.

Enough was enough as far as Kate was concerned. She dialled 999 and the paramedics were at the house within half an hour which I was grateful for. They found me looking like a draught excluder on the living room floor. When they realised there was no way I was getting up in the normal way, even with my arms around them, they tried one of their inflatable cushions, which are usually used to help old people from the floor after a fall.

'We've never had to pull this out for someone of your age before,' one of the paramedics joked, trying to keep the atmosphere light.

They managed to get me sat on the sofa, but the pain now was overwhelming. They strapped a mask over my face and started me on gas and air (nitrous oxide and oxygen). This enabled me to tolerate them standing me up and, with an arm wrapped around each of them, they tried to help me up to bed.

I wondered at the time why they weren't taking me to hospital, but the idea of being comfortable in my own bed was increasingly attractive, especially as the 'laughing gas' kicked in. We only lived in a small house with one flight of stairs. It was a journey that should take me forty seconds usually but, despite the pain relief, it took two hours to get me up to bed. Every couple of steps required a large dose of gas and air to get me through. I felt like a mountaineer in a storm near the summit of Everest, where the air is too thin to breathe properly. By the time I got to bed I had cleared the paramedics out of nitrous oxide.

I was high as a kite and finally in a position that I could tolerate (foetal with a pillow between my legs). The paramedics suggested I go to the toilet before I sleep, but I couldn't think about that. The pain when I moved, was just too much to bear, so they left me with a urine bottle which I could use from the bed at night if I needed it, and then they made to leave.

'Hang on!' I said anxiously. 'What do we do now? If it's not gone in the morning?'

'Well, it's difficult with back pain,' one of them sighed. 'We don't want to take you to A&E where you might have to wait in far less comfortable surroundings for a long time.'

'So?' Kate said.

'So, if things are not better in the morning, get in touch with your G.P.,' he smiled, and they were gone.

Kate looked doubtful, but they were the professionals, so I didn't think to question their approach. Besides, I was far too high to think straight.

TUESDAY

When I woke in the morning, the first thing I noticed was that I had wet the bed. I put it down to the fact that I was so off my head on gas and air last night that I'd lost all control. Unfortunately, the gas and air had long worn off and as I tried to shuffle out of the wet sheets, the pain returned with a vengeance.

It was clear to both Kate and I, that things had not got better at all, so she booked me an appointment at the G.P.

The surgery was only at the end of our road, a two-minute walk away, but there was no way I could walk there. Kate drove me to the door and after hobbling inside I saw a doctor who asked some questions and did a pin prick test. I still had good sensation in my legs during the test, but when the doctor tried to lift them, the pain was shocking.

The G.P. concluded that I had sciatica and prescribed amitriptyline, an antidepressant also used as a strong painkiller. I'd heard of sciatica and did my own googling on it when I got home. From what I read and what the doctor had said, I felt reassured that it might just be a matter of resting up until this particularly bad bout had gone away.

I called work and they signed me off for a while with *a bad back*. The drugs did their job and knocked me out, which was a relief, and I was able to sleep that night.

WEDNESDAY

Whenever I came round and tried to stretch, the pain was just as bad as before, if not worse.

I called the G.P. and told her. She suggested I wait another day to see if things settled. The thought of enduring this agony for another twenty-four long hours was too much to bear so I asked for more pain relief. The G.P. said I was on a particularly high dose of the amitriptyline already, but she agreed to add a little codeine to the mix to try to help me out.

Despite wielding the prescription from the doctor, the pharmacy refused to give it to me, stating I was already on enough painkillers and made me feel like a junkie trying to con them into giving me my next fix.

THURSDAY

Without my prescription fulfilled I had to find some other way to relieve this pain. My bladder and bowels were still functioning OK but standing up to wee was excruciating and sitting on the toilet was a painful process too. So, I booked an appointment with a chiropractor for the following morning.

FRIDAY

Unable to drive, my mum and stepfather drove me to the appointment. I'd read that acupuncture could help with sciatica, so I asked the chiropractor to stick a few pins in me while I was on her table. She began on my back. I'd never had acupuncture before, so I was relieved when the sensation of the pins going in wasn't painful. I could feel them as she stuck them in my lower back, my buttocks, then…

'Are you going to stick any in my legs?' I asked after a while.

'I already have,' she said.

She showed me how I resembled a hedgehog.

'Can't you feel them?' she asked.

I shook my head, dreading her response.

'I'm going to stop this session right now,' she said, 'and I advise you to go to A&E immediately.'

At A&E, when I explained that I was losing sensation in my legs, they moved me through for assessment quickly. They did a pin prick test and then a rectal examination was carried out. I remember not being able to feel all of the rectal examination – I didn't know whether to be worried or grateful that I couldn't feel the doctor's digits up my bum.

I was asked to pee in a pot, which was hard to do. I put that down to people coming in and out of the cubicle asking if I'd done it yet. The pressure to perform was intimidating. But eventually I managed it and then they took me for a scan which revealed there was some urine left in my bladder, something which there shouldn't be in someone of my age, I was told.

'That coupled with the lack of sensation in your legs and anus,' said a doctor, 'means we need to send you for an MRI straight away. And if you have what we think you have, we'll need to operate on you today.'

They didn't tell me what they thought I might have but I had gone from believing I had sciatica to possibly needing emergency surgery, and because we were in the middle of the pandemic, no one could even be with me.

I called my mum and my wife and told them what I'd been told. They were as incredulous as I was. I just had a bad back a few hours ago and now I was sitting alone in a poky little room waiting for the results of an MRI.

'Great news,' the junior doctor said as he strode in. 'It's not what we thought it was. We don't need to operate, and you can go home.'

Of course, it was a relief to hear that, but I still didn't know what was going on.

'Just rest up,' the doctor said. 'We'll sort you out with some crutches to help with the mobility until it gets better and plenty of painkillers too.'

Again, I had no reason to doubt nor question the professionals. So, I went home.

SATURDAY

I woke up as I'd woken up every morning for the past week. In agony.

SUNDAY

I was living a physically painful version of *Groundhog Day*.

That weekend felt like months. I was moving around like a *slug on the carpet,* according to my wife. I couldn't eat and I could barely speak as things got worse. It became more difficult to urinate. I would have to sit on the toilet and force it out. Sensation also lessened and by Sunday, I had lost all sensation in that area. Also, I had become quite constipated. I remember passing one bowel motion only on Sunday. Afterwards I couldn't feel anything when I wiped myself, that was different from a couple of days earlier, I am sure. I couldn't properly feel the rectal examination on Friday at A&E, but I could feel something; by Sunday I could feel nothing at all. The area of numbness increased over the weekend too. By Sunday the numbness in my left leg had spread and it felt as though it was all around my leg and down to the knee, whereas on Friday it had been just down the back of my left thigh.

Kate was furious that I'd never had a diagnosis from the hospital. 'I can't leave you here like this when I go to work tomorrow. This isn't safe. For you or the kids.'

'But what can we do?' I groaned. 'A&E sent me packing. The G.P. isn't open today.'

Kate thought for a moment then snapped her fingers. 'BUPA.'

'Eh?'

'You have private health insurance from work, don't you?'

'Oh yeah,' I said with a wince. It was just one of those perks we were given as employees of the bank. I'd never thought about using it.

'There's a private hospital in Bournemouth. Let's see if we can get you in there on your BUPA cover,' Kate said, picking up the phone.

MONDAY

That morning, a week after I first felt that awful pop, I was in the Nuffield telling a surgeon what had happened and how I had almost given up going to the toilet, as it was just too painful to push. The surgeon was very reassuring and guaranteed he would get to the root of what was going on that very day. I had another MRI and, minutes after, the surgeon was showing me the image they had taken.

'Look here, James,' he said indicating the base of the spine. 'A large part of this disc has herniated and is crushing the cauda equina nerves here. You have what's known as Cauda Equina Syndrome.'

'Cauda what?'

He pointed at an ominous dark patch on the scan. 'We should see all the cauda equina nerves here. They control your bladder, bowel, and leg function. We're seeing nothing as the herniated disc destroys them.'

Everything went hazy.

'When did you first go to hospital with this?' the surgeon asked.

'Friday,' I said, my voice trembling.

The surgeon shook his head. 'You should have been operated on then. The damage done already might be impossible to repair, but we need to operate right now, to try and avoid you being paralysed for the rest of your life.'

My heart sank. I could barely process what he was telling me. It was just sciatica, wasn't it? That's what the NHS hospital had suggested. 'Go home and rest', they said. My neighbour was waiting for me in the car park outside. He had dropped me off, as Kate had to go to work. I'd told him I'd be back in a few minutes after the scan. Now I was being told I might never walk again, and I was going under the knife… when?

'Right now,' said the surgeon.

I called my neighbour and told him what was happening. I called Kate barely able to talk sense through my tears.

'I'm coming,' she said.

'You can't,' I cried. 'COVID. They won't let anyone be with me.'

Suddenly everything went into fast-forward. Consent forms were put in front of me. I was told I had to call BUPA to get their authorisation for the Nuffield to do the operation. I was ringing around, searching for my membership number while the surgeon was coming in saying, 'We have to get that consent *now*. Are we covered to do it?'

I didn't know what I was doing. I'd never had to deal with insurance companies in this way before and certainly not while a surgeon was telling me the clock was ticking on the rest of my life.

After a nerve-wracking couple of calls, BUPA told me we were covered.

'Great, get your clothes off!' someone said.

And the next thing I knew I was on a trolley whizzing down the corridor into an operating theatre. I heard words like *decompression of the spine* and *L5-S1*. I nodded, as if I knew what the hell they were going on about. And then the anaesthetic did its job, and I went under.

***

I woke up in a comfortable looking room.

In a daze I looked down and saw a tube coming out of my penis attached to a bag full of urine on the side of the bed.

'What the...?'

'Hi James,' smiled the surgeon. 'The operation was a success.'

He showed me a clear pot in which was a chunk of spinal disc with bits of pink flesh hanging off, of it. 'This is what we removed from your back. This was the stuff that was crushing your cauda equina nerves. How's the pain?' he asked knowingly.

I thought about it for a moment and then confirmed what he clearly suspected. 'It's gone,' I smiled. 'You're a genius. Thank you so much,' I gasped with relief. 'You're a miracle worker. That's…'

'Well,' he stopped me before I got too excited. 'I've relieved the pressure to stop things getting any worse, but because this wasn't picked up earlier, this,' he said waving the pot at me, 'has been killing off the nerves for a few days and now I think you'll have trouble with your bladder and your bowels, perhaps even your sexual function.'

My face dropped.

'Did you have issues with sex in the days before you came here?'

'Um…' I said distractedly. 'Sex was the last thing on my mind for the past week, doctor.'

He nodded sympathetically, then said, 'Well, it's key that we get you mobile as quickly as possible before the brain disassociates with those damaged nerves. It'll take some retraining of the bladder and bowels. But be warned, it could be up to two years before we really know just how much recovery you'll be able to make and what the rest of your life will look like.'

I was on a rollercoaster of emotions again. Two minutes ago, I was virtually dancing about in my bed with joy and now I felt as if I was in the dock being handed down a prison sentence. Two years, with no chance of parole.

I called Kate and told her the news; the news that I might not be able to walk properly ever again, that I might need a catheter for the rest of my life and getting an erection might be out of the question. There were so many unknowns and so many fears, I felt as if I was staring into darkness, fumbling and faltering forward.

They kept me in the Nuffield for seven days. Due to COVID, no one but Kate was allowed in to see me and even then, she had to be masked and gowned and visored and we couldn't sit near each other, let alone hug. I would sit in a wheelchair by the window as she drove the kids and my mum into the car park so we could wave to each other through the glass and speak on the phone. I felt like a caged animal. I didn't know who I was anymore.

I didn't feel lucky at the time, but a physio started work with me immediately while I was in the Nuffield, a service which I don't think I would have got, certainly not so quickly, in an NHS hospital.

I had to use crutches to try and walk – a nice shiny set made for someone as tall as me and a sharp contrast to the busted old set the NHS hospital gave me, which would have only suited a hobbit – but I could only manage half of the corridor before I lost control.

We then tried the stairs, but I couldn't step up with my left foot. It felt like a dead weight. I had no feeling in it.

'I just want to step up,' I cried. 'Why can't I do it?'

My whole life I had been active and able, and I had just taken that for granted. I thought of Freddie again. My toddler might be walking properly before I can. What the hell! I felt so embarrassed.

'Am I paralysed?' I said to the physio.

'Partially yes,' he said honestly, 'but if we keep repeating these exercises we can try and get those signals working in the nerves again.'

After a week, my time in private care had run out, so I was transferred to the Salisbury NHS hospital where they had a spinal unit. I was nervous, about leaving the safe haven of private care. I googled Duke of Cornwall Spinal Centre Salisbury and read a lot of good reviews about the spinal unit, which reassured me. There, I was told, I would continue my rehabilitation which might take they said up to twelve weeks.

They allowed Kate to drive me to Salisbury to give us a chance to be together again, however briefly. But I hardly said a word on the journey. Kate described me after, as a lost soul. I was just staring at my now useless feet, or looking at the world rushing past the window, everyone going about their lives apparently without a care in the world. People hopping on and off of buses, running up the street, walking with their loved ones, laughing, joking, normal stuff, all of which I could do last week.

As we entered the unit, I could see different people in wheelchairs shuffling around, some with limbs missing. I wanted to tell the nurses I must be in the wrong place. I wasn't like them. Was I?

After checking in at reception, Kate began carrying my bags towards the ward, but she was stopped halfway down the corridor.

'You can't go in,' she was told by a nurse.

'I beg your pardon?' Kate said indignantly.

'COVID,' the nurse explained. 'And James, you must go into this isolation room until you've had two negative COVID tests, then you can go onto the ward.'

Isolated from my wife, isolated from other patients, I had that sense of being jailed again. I was assessed as I had been on that first night in A&E. Various people coming in and out of the room. Pricked with pins, fingers up my arse. I felt violated but found myself apologising for not being able to feel anything in my left leg.

They tried me without a catheter, and I wet the bed, so they asked me to try putting in a catheter myself, giving me video tutorials to watch. I really struggled to do this, not just physically, but emotionally. I couldn't believe that I needed this contraption inside me to do something as simple as pass urine.

The physio would come in and try and get me doing various exercises which I found really hard. I got so frustrated with my inability to do simple movements. And when staff weren't coming in and out, I had nothing to do but stew on my situation, brood on all the things I could no longer do.

I would FaceTime my wife and kids and get them to drive into the car park, which my little isolation room looked out onto. Without seeing them, even just through the glass, I would never have coped. The rest of the time I spent googling Cauda Equina Syndrome, frantically searching for some sort of answer or miracle cure.

That's when I stumbled across Cauda Equina Champions Charity. I saw there was a support group and a helpline. I had felt so isolated so far that I requested a call back and, in a short space of time, Claire phoned me.

Speaking to someone who had experienced what I was going through was priceless. I had a million and one questions, and she was prepared to answer them all. I started to speak to other members of the group. I didn't really want to speak to anyone else in the outside world anymore, only people I could relate to, people who had gone through what I was going through. All my friends and family would send messages, wishing me well, telling me that now the operation was a *success* I'd be back to normal soon. They had the best of intentions, and I was so grateful to be in their thoughts, but they didn't really understand that I would never be *back to normal*. And the idea of being stuck in this unit for twelve weeks was so depressing I didn't have the will to explain this to them.

As much as I didn't want to be in the rehab unit a second longer, I didn't want to go home and have Kate and the kids see me like I was: half the man I used to be. I felt trapped, useless, and felt myself going to a very dark place; the kind of place where you consider taking your own life. The last time I felt like that, I realised, was when my dad died.

And it was then that he came to mind.

That smiling face of his, that Blitz spirit. 'Keep going, son! Push on through!' he would say if he were here now. To him, family was everything. To me, family was everything too. And I could hear him telling me I had to fight for my family as much as for myself. I scrolled through photos of my kids and Kate, of us together on those happy holidays, all those memories we'd made, and I thought about all the memoires yet to be made. It was a bit of a lightbulb moment for me. I *had* to get better and out of here. And the only way I knew to get better at anything was to set goals.

I did it in my work life. I would set development goals and I would make it my business to smash them – that's how I rose through the ranks so quickly at such a young age. I also did it when I went running. One mile turned into two and before I knew it, I was doing a 10K and a half marathon. The same must apply here, I thought. And just as when I would post on social media about how many miles I'd ran, I felt the best way to explain to friends and family the reality of my condition, was to post about Cauda Equina Syndrome and the goals I had set myself. After all, what else did I have to do stuck in this isolation room all day?

Cauda Equina Champions Charity was quickly becoming a cause close to my heart and so I decided to start a fundraiser for them to accompany my posts.

The first goal I set myself was to learn to use these bloody catheters properly on my own, and when I did it, I posted proudly that I could. I wrote about my dark times and how I had taken my physical health for granted all these years and it really seemed to resonate with people online. The response was overwhelmingly positive and the fundraiser soon topped its original £150 goal and ended up bringing in £1400 for the charity and more importantly, knowledge about the condition to those who assumed I would be fine soon enough.

After one long week in isolation, I was testing negative for COVID and was moved onto the ward. Meeting and being able to chat to other people, was a joy. I was in group physio sessions every other day and the rest of the time I was doing exercises by myself, trying to smash my latest goal and get out of this place, before the twelve weeks I had been given.

I started to feel like I was gaining some control over my bladder again and, determined to be free of catheters, I went to the toilet one day and pushed and pushed to get the urine out without a device attached to me. The result was that I started to bleed quite heavily from the penis. I had overdone it. And it was a reminder to not rush my recovery. Little wins were what it was all about again. Little wins that could add up to one big triumph.

Listening to the doctors, I started to record all my fluid intake and output and think about retraining my mindset when it came to going to the toilet. I learnt a lot about my condition and passed what I was learning onto my followers on social media.

One area I hadn't thought about too much was sexual function, but the doctors now asked me to think seriously about this. I was offered various types of Viagra to try out, but at first my male pride got in the way.

'I'm on a ward with three other men,' I told the doctors wryly. 'They're lovely blokes, but in the middle of the night most of us are having our bowels evacuated or we're wetting the bed. I don't think it's exactly the right environment for me to get an erection.'

Trying to keep things light, I would post about this on social media and so my mates would send me NSFW messages on our WhatsApp group chats. *Perhaps this'll help*, they wrote with a wink emoji or two.

…but no cigar.

I put it down to the environment again to keep myself from getting disheartened, but the nurses said they would send me home with some Viagra and a vacuum pump just in case.

After just three weeks, the doctors were happy for me to go home. I was elated. I cried even more that day than when my children were born. I felt like I was getting out of jail, but at the same time I was sad to say goodbye to my fellow 'inmates.' We had formed a little family of our own in there. We spent every waking moment together and we would push each other to achieve our goals. When one of us was having a bad day the rest of us would take the slack and encourage him to keep going. The world we had known had been put on hold. Before my injury I was all about career, promotion, life moving at break-neck speeds, trying to cram everything in. Now I and my fellow patients were just taking one day at a time. Refocusing. Finding new perspectives and priorities.

When I left, I was sent on my way with catheters, suppositories, and erection aids. I felt like Lily leaving one of her friend's birthday parties, but the contents of my goodie bag were slightly different to hers. The sweeties inside my bag were Amitriptyline, Tramadol, Oramorph for pain and Sertraline as an antidepressant, to name but a few. These had all been spoon fed to me by the nurses on the ward every day. Now I had to be responsible for what dose I was taking and when. It was a little daunting to be honest.

Back home I was in floods of tears again at the welcome home banners and my family all around me, who I could touch and hug for the first time in a month. I walked the length of the hallway with my crutches. I was shaky but that was a far cry from the last time I was here.

The staircase, however, loomed above me like a climbing wall. In the spinal unit, nearly everything was on one level and if not, we had lifts to get up and down. Kate was here now to help me up the stairs, but when I got to the bathroom, I was all fingers and thumbs when it came to using my catheters again. I was gutted. I felt like I had gone backwards in my recovery. But Kate was my greatest cheerleader. She reminded me that it was just a matter of adjusting to this new environment. I could do it. Little wins.

It was also tough when my kids would say, 'Are you better? Can we play with you now?'

I had to explain that it would be many months before I was able to lift the smallest of things, let alone a young human.

They also had questions when they saw me preparing a suppository in the bathroom. 'Daddy, what is that? Why are you sticking it up your bum?'

At first, I was embarrassed, but I knew it wouldn't help to hide things from them, so I explained what a suppository was for, why I used a catheter and why I couldn't bend down easily.

Kate bought me a long-handled claw to help me with the bending part and I soon realised that the most reassuring thing to do for the kids was involve them in everything; make a game of it even. Freddie was obsessed with my claw so we bought one for him too and every time he saw me pick something up that I had dropped he would do the same with his dinosaurs and toy cars which littered the house. Suddenly my condition wasn't so alien to him and we had a tidy house! It was a win-win.

Kate was supported by her employers, they stopped her on call and night shifts so she could be there for the kids. She was also allowed to stay home for the first few weeks so we could get used to a life which was new to us all. Friends helped drop the kids off and pick them up from school, everyone was revolving around me.

And it made me feel guilty.

We couldn't rely on the goodwill of friends and family forever, but nothing was changing significantly in terms of my recovery. How long was this going to go on for?

My employers had granted me full pay for six months while I got better so I could continue to keep my new focus and concentrate on getting fitter, but the six-month cut off point was soon coming over the horizon. After that I would be on half-pay and then there would be no way we could pay the mortgage. I was keen to go back to work, but I didn't know how it would be possible with my constant fatigue, toilet needs and the practicalities of getting around the old bank building with its countless stairs. Once again, I felt like half the man I used to be. HR would need to begin a medical assessment to see if I was fit to come back to work and there was talk of being retired from my role if the adaptions I needed, were not possible for the bank to make.

Yet at the same time in early 2021 the bank, like many employers in the post-COVID world, were realising the need to streamline their workforces and save money, so redundancies among the management team were imminent. When I heard this, I wondered whether I should take redundancy myself to really focus on my physical and mental health. A redundancy pay-out could keep me going for another year, which would take me close to the two years my surgeon had told me was needed to fully realise the extent of my recovery.

I took the redundancy.

I spent my time working with a physio, attending hydrotherapy sessions, which helped enormously, and I didn't have to worry about where the next penny was coming from. I was found myself in a much better pace mentally, perhaps more so than I had been in years.

During those six months off work, I had filled some of my spare time by acting as a volunteer for Cauda Equina Champions Charity. Since my first effort at fundraising in that isolation room had gone so well, I had been taken on to do more fundraising and it really gave me something to focus on, something close to my heart, something which also helped my recovery mentally.

Later in 2021, Claire had become a very good friend and I was loving my time volunteering for the charity. That's when Claire asked me if I wanted a permanent position at the organisation. It made perfect sense. I loved the work, I valued the support I got from them concerning my condition, I valued the help I could be to others, and what better employer could someone with Cauda Equina Syndrome have than a charity that specialises in it and fully understands the challenges people with it face every day?

Consequently, I started working for the charity from home on a part time basis and if I was having a bad day because of the CES, Claire would know exactly what I was going through. She knew it wasn't because I was hungover or trying to pull a sickie. She got it. And that is priceless in a world that still has little comprehension of the impact CES has on people's lives.

By July 2021 I was working alongside Claire at the charity, my managerial skills from the bank proving to be an asset. I found myself delivering presentations on CES to hospital staff and medical students, educating them so that one day they might not overlook a CES patient as the A&E doctors once overlooked me. And now I'm helping new members navigate this sea of change in their lives, as Claire once helped me in my darkest hour.

Despite still suffering the aftermath of CES, my friends and family tell me I've never looked happier. And they're right. I feel a huge sense of satisfaction from my work now and don't carry the same weight on my shoulders that I did at the bank, a burden which I took home with me, and which kept me from spending enough time with my family.

Now I have the ideal work-life balance and I am there for my kids in a way I couldn't be before. We're certainly worse off financially than we were before, but we're richer in happiness. We know we took our health for granted before and now we make it our priority, because no amount of money can buy physical and mental wellbeing.

I still am unable to walk great distances and running is out of the question. I miss that so much, that sense of my body rushing through the air, that sense of being able to compete, that adrenaline rush. It was one of the things that kept me referring disparagingly to myself as *half the man I used to be*.

My wife's cousin, who happens to be a physio, pointed me in the direction of many other sports, apart from running, that are available to the disabled.

Disabled.

That was a new way of referring to myself that I had to get my head around, but it was a lot more positive than *half the man I used to be*. I was a whole person, a whole person with a disability. And once I had flicked that switch in my brain, I could start to explore my options.

Although these days I use a crutch to get around sometimes and only need a wheelchair to get myself over long distances, I found myself joining a wheelchair rugby team and embracing my disability rather than hiding from it. I had such fun playing rugby that I now play every Sunday and have found myself rubbing shoulders with so many inspiring people and great disabled sportsmen and women.

Two years on from my injury, I have to accept, that things now are pretty much the way they might be forever. My mobility has improved – I walk intermittently with crutches and on long distances I use a wheelchair – but I still need set alarms to remind me to go to the toilet with the aid of a catheter and suppositories as my bladder and bowels still don't tell me when they're full. My sexual function is non-existent and that led to some guilt where Kate was concerned. Not only could I not satisfy her in that department, but she was always helping me around the house when I wanted to help myself and couldn't. It made me snappy, which was totally out of character, but I was so frustrated that I couldn't simply pick the kids up in my arms or pick a pen up off the floor. Kate would never complain about helping me, but I'd see her getting tired and so, feeling sorry for myself, I'd tell her she didn't have to stay with me. Surely it was too much to ask.

Luckily, Kate didn't take me up on that offer and I started counselling to help me deal with the depression, just like I did when Dad passed away. We came through it all stronger than ever.

Every day is a challenge now, but I can't say any two days are the same – it's certainly not boring. We are all adapting to the 'new norm' and not taking life for granted. We have a great support network of family and friends, who now understand my condition and continuously offer help where possible to make our lives that little bit easier. Special mention to our parents and sisters: Teresa, Phil, Carrie, Kev, Caroline, Emily, and Alice.

We're making more time for each other and the kids than we ever did in the past and we're making memories like never before.

I will be forever grateful to my spinal surgeon for all the care and support he gave me throughout this challenging time in my life. Without his instant diagnosis, it is almost certain that I would be permanently paralysed.

CATRINA'S STORY

Falling in love with my wheelchair.

Margot Fonteyn was my idol.

She was revered by many for her elegance and lyricism, but what I related to was what some criticised in her: her lack of formal technique as she moved across the floor without rigidity, with a body that wasn't a stereotypically perfect ballerina's shape but still incredibly beautiful. Her flair and her passion were indisputable. Her personality always shone through in every performance and her movement was captivating. She didn't conform and I related to that.

As a child I tried Irish dancing at first, but I found its strict form quite difficult to attune to. Dancing came naturally to me, but the technique required in some disciplines was restrictive to the way my body yearned to move. I just wanted to dance in my own way. So, I kept trying different styles: ballet, contemporary, jazz, looking for something that suited me.

When I danced, I was transported to another place. It was a place of great solace for me because there, I could forget for a while about all the awful things that were happening to my dad.

He had cancer and was so ill. I knew I needed to help my mum. It broke my heart to see his decline and the effect it was having on her. I was only nine at the time, but my efforts were noticed by a neighbour who nominated me for a Child of Achievement Award.

The ceremony was at the Queen Elizabeth Conference Centre on the banks of the Thames in London and had all the glitz and glamour you would expect, TV news cameras, celebrity guests and the Prime Minister himself, John Major. But my favourite part of the whole experience was when my parents and I went out to get some air and walked along the river to see the Houses of Parliament. Just the three of us, away from all the intensity of the award ceremony. It was my first time seeing this iconic place and it took my breath away. I stood there, open-mouthed dreaming of one day living in London and working in parliament.

There was an ice cream van nearby, so we bought a 99 each, and as we sat outside in the winter sun, I thought how lucky I was.

'You know why you came into our lives?' my dad said.

I shook my head.

'You came along so your mum would always have someone to dance with.'

I knew my dad was still very ill. I knew he was implying that he wouldn't be around much longer to dance with Mum. I wasn't ready to hear that, but the memory of that moment I treasure because what he said proved to be very true, despite everything that would happen to me in the following decade.

A year later to the day my dad died at home surrounded with love; with my brother Damian, my Mum and me. I will never forget that day. The only way I could deal with the devastation I felt, was to throw myself into dance. I lived and breathed dance to such an extent that by the age of fifteen I was teaching my own dance class and competing at world class levels.

I found a home in the Modern Linedance style. This is a form of dance which is an amalgamation of many styles from ballroom to Latin. My mum would take me to competitions on weekends. I'd dance three or four times a week and on Monday evenings I would teach both adults and children at a working men's club in Oxenhope, near my home in West Yorkshire. Doing everything by the book: I took a Best Western Dance Academy teacher training course and my family helped with insurance and public playing licenses.

However, I experienced more loss when more relatives were taken away from me. I lost my aunt and my grandmother in the few years after my dad, but the dance community was a second family to me and brought so much joy into my life, that it eased the effects of the grief.

My godson Finn was born when I was just fourteen. He was the son of my Mum's close friends, who used to take me in after school sometimes when Dad was particularly ill, or Mum was working. Finn's sister Mya and I grew up like sisters. When Finn came along, I loved him so much as if he was my own family. They all *are* my family in my heart. Unexpectedly, when Finn was born, he had Down's Syndrome. This drew me to him in ways I couldn't quite understand at the time but would become clear later in my life. Being a godmother to him, an aunt to the nieces and nephews my three older brothers had blessed me with, and being a dancer were the things that defined me. I lived for those things.

When I was seventeen, a couple of days prior to the World Dance Masters Championship, as I worked hard on my routines, my back froze, and I found myself struggling to move. I saw a physio who said I needed to rest completely and questioned whether I should take part in the competition at all. Missing the championship was out of the question as far as I was concerned and so with a combination of heat and ice and laying down in the dressing area of the Winter Garden Ballroom until the very moment I had to go on the dancefloor, I not only got through it, but I won.

The pain didn't subside, however, and after my win I had an MRI which showed I had a degenerative disease of the discs in my spine, one of which was partially prolapsed.

Determined not to let that stop me following my dreams, I went to the University of Roehampton to study dance. I had watched the movie *Fame,* over and over again, since I was a child, and I dreamed that my college dancing days would be something like that.

Actually… they were better.

I was disappointed when I started having back problems again and had to have a year out after my first year. But I came back stronger in the second and third years and had the time of my life. I joined a theatre group on campus where I made lifelong friends and in my final year, I choreographed *Return to the Forbidden Planet* and found that choreography was something I really wanted to focus on. Through choreography I was keen to guide dancers away from the rigidity of form and towards musicality; making sure that dance was a response to the music and not something merely technical and separate from sound.

I once again threw myself headfirst into the show, rehearsing most nights and then dancing through my classes all day. However, that took its toll on my body. After the show was done, I started to have even more serious back pain than before, and I had to have a microdiscectomy. This is an operation where some of the disc, which was protruding in my spine and compressing the spinal nerve root, was taken away to relieve the pressure on the nerves, which were causing pain in my legs.

This meant that I couldn't finish all the physical requirements of my course and I left Roehampton with an

HND rather than the full degree and my dreams of being a professional dancer dissolving fast.

As I considered my future, a great friend suggested I might enjoy working as a teaching assistant. They were so right. I loved working with children as much as I loved being an aunt, and it wasn't long before I was teaching a dance class at the local school in the afternoons, and in the mornings. I was supporting a wonderful young girl with Down's Syndrome. I was drawn to her like I was to my godson, and it soon became clear that I didn't just need dance in my life, but I also needed to feel that I was of service to people with disabilities, each of these different aspects of my day nourishing the different facets of my soul.

Life was good. I was even in a good place with my ex-boyfriend Luke and his family. We had remained good friends and one autumn weekend we had booked to go on a trip to London to see an American football match at Wembley. We would be staying at the Hilton on Park Lane, so everything was set for a fun trip away.

I was on a high when my team, the Chicago Bears, won the game against Tampa Bay, but before we left the stadium, I simply bent down to pick up my handbag and felt something in my back go. The discomfort was enormous, but I had had plenty of back problems before, so I assumed it was more of the same. I didn't make a fuss at the time because I didn't want to ruin the weekend that was going so well, but when I woke in the morning in the hotel room the pain in my back and down my legs was excruciating and now, to add to my problems, I couldn't go to the toilet. Luke suggested we call an ambulance, but there was no way I was going to do that. We were in the Hilton! I could just imagine what a scene that would make. I would have been so embarrassed, and then if we had got to the hospital and it was nothing, I would have looked like either a fool or a drama queen.

I wanted to look strong, but in the end the pain was just too much to bear, and Luke persuaded me to go to hospital in a taxi. He stayed with me as I was triaged and we waited for an MRI after which I was told I would have to have an operation the next morning, because I had a condition called Cauda Equina Syndrome.

Luke called my Mum, and I was prepped for surgery. My best friends Terri and Keely came when Luke had to leave, and Mum arrived that night. In the morning I was transferred to Guys Hospital. I was seen by the anaesthetist and was told I was first on the list that morning, but just before I was taken to theatre, the consultant in charge decided that I didn't need surgery after all and, since I was relatively young at twenty-three and hadn't been involved in a major trauma, the condition could be treated 'conservatively.'

So, I was put on a ward for a week and given plenty of painkillers and some physio, but that seemed to be it. The doctor who had made the initial diagnosis of CES visited me frequently and seemed keen for me to still get the surgery asking the consultant to reassess me, but the doctor was consistently overruled by his superior, who never saw me again after the five minutes he spent with me. There was clearly a difference of opinion between them but that just left me in a cloud of confusion and anxiety in an environment I didn't want to be in, especially because I didn't really understand what good it was doing to keep me in the hospital.

When the week was up, I was allowed to go home. But as soon as I did, the CES manifested fully and unequivocally this time. I was operated on the following day and was left with severe issues with walking, bladder and bowel control and all the typical symptoms of CES.

But I believed I wasn't going to be the typical CES sufferer.

I would be OK, I told myself. This thing wouldn't take over my life. I would get up on my crutches and get back to work straight away.

Some members of my family talked about people they knew who lived perfectly content lives and used wheelchairs. So, they said, why couldn't I? But I didn't want them to ever think I wasn't trying. I wanted them to be proud of me, to believe I was working hard, making enough effort with my physio, striving to get better. It felt like I was continually striving for this perfect recovery for them, but I kept falling short.

I don't think anyone had an idea about the kind of physical pain I was enduring, and they also didn't know the kind of mental anguish I was facing because I had lost the ability to have full movement and control over my body, something that was so intrinsic to my life, to who I was, to my sense of self when my identity was so inextricably linked to dance. My love of being of service to children with learning disabilities, another facet of myself that was so important to me, was also threatened by this condition. What use was I in this world if I couldn't even help others?

I felt as if I was grieving once more.

I had grieved for my dad, my gran, my aunt and now I felt a loss like that again. But instead of admitting that to myself or telling my family or friends how much I was struggling, I gave the impression I was fine. I was strong. I could defeat this thing and so I powered on, determined to do the impossible. I tried to fill the hole in my life and my sense of being no use to anyone by buying people gifts to make up for my physical absence, but there was never a gift good enough to make up for how I felt.

I decided to set up a website called Secrets of a Beauty Addict. I used the platform to talk about art, beauty standards, cosmetics, pop culture and raise awareness for charities. It did quite well; I even started interviewing people I admired like Katie Piper, Kye Sones and Daniel Sandler. I tried to reach people with positivity and light using what I had to hand: my laptop from my bed. I wanted to help make people feel better about themselves. I wanted to make myself feel better too and it spawned a love of writing in me, giving me a platform for my poetry that later became a vehicle to express my disability. Plus, the PR packages were incredible!

Within a year though, I had another episode of CES.

This time my legs were affected so severely there was no denying I had to use a wheelchair and my bladder function was impaired to an even greater extent than before. Intermittent catheterization was not working for me anymore and so it became necessary for me to have a suprapubic catheter, one that is fixed surgically to the bladder through a hole made just below the navel and leads to a large bag which I carry around in a backpack on my chair.

On the plus side I had a wonderful consultant this time, who seemed to have great empathy for my situation. He understood the impact the CES was having on my life. He took the time to make sure I knew exactly what was happing regarding my condition and gave me hope for the future. He advised me that I needed what's known as a TLIF surgery, or to give it its full name: transforaminal lumbar interbody fusion. This would be the best way he told me, to prevent me getting yet another episode of Cauda Equina Syndrome or any other compression on the spinal cord further up, which I was prone to due to the degenerative disc disease and the fact that I had always been hypermobile – this had once been an asset to me as a dancer, but now added to the risk of more problems in future.

Despite my consultant's best efforts, the operation didn't work in the way we had hoped, the fusion failed and so I had to have another more extensive fusion of my spine.

I didn't think there was a greater pain than having Cauda Equina Syndrome, but the pain I felt as I came around from the anaesthetic after that second fusion surgery topped it. I had just endured a nine-hour operation, but I spent another two hours in resuscitation while the doctors tried to stabilize me. I can only assume that because of all the pain medication I had taken over the four or five years since my first episode of CES, I had built up a tolerance to the painkillers they gave me as I was coming round. Through the haze of grogginess, I could make out the faces of doctors and nurses I didn't know rushing around and looking worried. I could hear someone screaming and screaming and screaming… and then I realised it was me. And then I saw my mum's face clearly in front of me, speaking calmly and soothingly. She had been waiting in the hospital chapel during my surgery and the doctors had asked her to come to the resuscitation room when they saw how much I was suffering. It was the best medicine I could have had right then. I concentrated with all my might on her expression, and her touch was a balm like no other. Despite her efforts, my pain was still so incredibly intense that the doctors resorted to giving me ketamine and finally the pain was under control.

Life became more home-based after that. I needed hoisting from my bed and so we had carers come in to help with some of my personal care. We also had a stairlift installed in the house, which was generously paid for by SSAFA the armed forces charity, since my dad had been in the Royal Air Force.

I had to admit defeat, as far as going back to work was concerned, but took on a number of projects that I could do from the living room, such as making cards with one of my close friends Ruth, who was a continual support. And when my other friends, who had all been having babies over recent years, came to visit and keep me company, I would do activities with the little ones as if I was back working at the local school. This brought me so much joy, especially reading to them. I bought a changing mat and a baby bath, all the things that my friends would need when they brought the kids round, so they didn't have to think twice about coming.

But then things got bad again.

Every time I so much as sat up in bed I would be sick or faint. I tried to see my friends as before, but eventually I had to remain lying down in bed.

I stayed inside for the next sixteen months, rarely being able to get out of bed. I would make it downstairs occasionally for a change of scenery to say hi to friends, but within a half hour or so I would be feeling nauseous and would have to make my apologies before getting back to bed.

The symptoms were most probably caused, the doctors said, by a CSF (cerebrospinal fluid) leak, but no one seemed to be sure. And, if it was a leak, where was it was coming from? The only surgeons with the resources and expertise to help me were based in California. After so many months in bed, I became more and more vacant and confused, so my amazing friends Amy and Jenny led a fundraiser and eventually with the help of family, friends and my community we found the cash to fly me to L.A.

Finn's mother Gerry, who was a nurse, accompanied Mum and I on our journey to get the CSF leak patched and after yet another surgery was performed on me in America, I was happy to be able to sit up without wanting to vomit. My head no longer throbbed, and my thoughts were not so jumbled anymore.

It was a joy to spend time with my close friend Heather, who came to stay with us in LA as I recovered. And when I returned home to Yorkshire three weeks later, I was not only thinking straight, but I felt a fundamental shift in perspective and my outlook on life. I had spent so much time confined to my bed, that now I was just grateful to be breathing in fresh air and feeling the sun on my face. I had spent so much time after Cauda Equina Syndrome pushing myself to be the person I was before, and to do all the things that I could do before, but now I realised that I wasn't the same person and I had to begin embracing life in a different way.

Before I'd been confined to my bed, I had been going to pain management courses. I read every book I could find on the science of pain, I tried acupuncture, craniosacral therapy and if someone spoke about something that helped them with pain, I would try that too. But the method I relied on most of all was to just pretend the pain wasn't there.

Then I came across the Cauda Equina Champions Charity, and I learnt through the Breathworks course I accessed through them, that what I needed to do first was acknowledge the pain, then find out what it was that I needed to help me live with it. I still use medication now, but I think I have a more balanced view of it and am very aware at all times of just how much medication I am using.

I saw how people like Claire at the charity lived *with* their CES and not *against* it. Instead of trying to be the person I was before and trying to live in the same way, Claire taught me that if I wanted to go to work, for example, it was OK to ask for reasonable adjustments to the workplace to help me function in the way I now needed to. I didn't need to struggle on crutches as I was still tried to do. My legs were so heavy, quick to fatigue and lacking in sensation that a wheelchair was necessary most of the time and that, she made me understand, was OK; it wasn't failure, as I once thought it was. I didn't need to hide away. The outside world would have to get used to and accommodate the new me as much as I would.

Suddenly I realised that my chair could take me to places my body couldn't. It enabled me. It opened doors. The grief I had felt in my young life, losing my dad, my aunt and gran, had taught me from a young age that life was finite. It had left a ticking clock in my mind that had spurred me on to push myself to achieve in ways which, post-CES, were sometimes counterproductive. So, having been bedridden for so long and not knowing then if I would ever get out of bed again, I knew now that there wasn't another moment to lose. I was going to seize every one of those moments. And my chair would help me do that.

That's how I fell in love with my wheelchair.

Champions Charity had been so helpful to me that with my newfound perspective I wanted to give something back to them. So, I started to volunteer for the charity and my world opened up even more. I discovered skills I didn't know I had. I started off in charge of the social media strategy with the skills I'd learned from my website, but soon found myself presenting to groups to help raise funding and speaking to the media on behalf of the charity.

After one item I did for BBC News I was trolled hideously. I had gone from being a dancer with a body like Margot Fonteyn, to having a much more sedentary lifestyle in the chair, so inevitably I had put on some pounds. But the insidious comments about my weight came thick and fast. And one poor soul commented:

```
        Somebody should put a knife to your
throat. You'd cost a lot less to the NHS
                   then.
```

Yes, *a poor soul*. I thought long and hard about it and I concluded they must have been in a very dark place to write such a thing. I replied:

```
        I really hope you find some light
in your life. You must have been feeling
 very low to write what you wrote. I've
been in a dark place too, but I hope you
 feel even some of the gratitude towards
life that I feel every morning now. I'm
          truly rooting for you.
```

Just as I could empathise with the 'troll', I found huge fulfilment in being able to speak to other people with CES; to tell them my truth and make them understand that I was not just offering tea and sympathy, but I was down there in the trenches, with them on their journey; and most importantly, that there was a way out of the darkness.

It was during one of my meetings for the charity with a company that supplies catheters, that I mentioned to the rep Harriet, that I used to be a dancer.

'Ooh, do you watch *Strictly*?' she asked.

'No, no, I can't,' I told her. 'I would struggle to watch other people dancing when I can't anymore, you know.'

She nodded and after we spoke a bit more she said, 'Actually I know someone at Northern Ballet. And they have this inclusive course there called In Motion. Do you fancy it?'

I had pretty much pushed dance away from my life and focused on helping others after my epiphany in L.A., but it was that very same epiphany, that shift in mental attitude, that told me to seize every opportunity that came my way; and here was an opportunity being handed to me on a plate. Saying no wouldn't feed that spirit that was nourishing me so well these days, would it? So, I said:

'Yes,' and smiled at Harriet. 'Why not?'

The day came for the session at Northern Ballet. I was apprehensive. I feared it might be a trainwreck. I feared physical pain and a dent to my mental wellbeing.

When I arrived, I was told I could get out of my beloved wheelchair and into a different one. It was a wheelchair specially designed for dance: super lightweight, thin wheels to increase speed, without so much back support so you feel like you have full range of motion, and, as you become more skilled, you can experiment with gravity and that new range of motion you have in the chair. The experience is a lot more intuitive than being in your average chair.

To me it felt like flying.

It was incredible. It was painful for my body at first, but for my soul it was transformative. That feeling I had had when I danced as a child, when all the horrible things were forgotten for a while, that same feeling came over me when I danced now. I was not just at one with the music, I *was* the music and I soared.

I made new friends that day and met people who knew my old friends. There was a sense of fate about the whole thing. There were people on the course who could move nothing more than a few fingers, people with cerebral palsy, some in electric wheelchairs. I knew more than ever that it was a gift that I could move any part of my body, and the sense of inclusion for everyone on that course was exemplary.

On the way home I cried. I felt a maelstrom of emotions, but the tears, I think, were mainly happy ones.

Not long after that wonderful session I started to develop something not so wonderful. Autonomic dysreflexia. Some people with spinal cord injuries develop this. You may have lost feeling and muscle control below the damaged spot, but the nerves there still try to send signals back to the brain, which can make your body do the wrong thing. So, something pinching my leg for example, might not be registered by my brain as that, but instead it would affect my breathing or my heart rate and could result in a stroke, seizure, or heart attack. So, I was prescribed a GTN spray, which people with angina spray under their tongues to stop chest pain and cardiac arrest.

I pulled back from my volunteering for a while as I needed to get a handle on this new issue that had been thrown at me, but I continued volunteering for an organisation that works with people with learning disabilities called People First Keighley & Craven, which was closer to home. I later became a permanent employee there in the role of Health Campaigner and more recently was successful in my application for the Team Leader position.

It's my dream job.

I have a wonderful boss who says, 'We don't make excuses, we make adjustments.' She and Claire from Champions Charity have inspired me to dream big and focus on solutions not problems.

As I look back over my life now, I realise this was where I was headed the whole time. Through my work with People First, I started running dance classes for people with learning disabilities and autism through an initiative with MENCAP called Round The World in co-production with Keighley Healthy Living. And most recently my role has involved working with groups such as The Mental Diversity Law Network along with Dr Lucy Series creating an accessible workshop regarding the current changes to The Human Rights Act with specific attention to the changes to the Deprivation of Liberty Safeguards. A job in the Houses of Parliament might not be so far away after all.

I am busier than ever, and I have never been happier, even in the days before I had a disability.

I hate the notion that I *needed* to go through what I've been through to come to this point of contentment and if anyone had said such a thing when I was in hospital on all those occasions, I would have been furious with them for what sounds like such rubbish. I wouldn't wish the pain I went through on anyone, and there are many different paths in life that *might* have led me to this point too, but it was my journey through CES that has left me happier than before it. And in that sense alone, I needed it.

So many people with learning disabilities don't always have all the words at their disposal to communicate how they feel, and I believe strongly that dance can give such people a powerful means of expression. The technique is not important. Just as I felt when I found Irish dance and ballet so daunting as a child, all I needed to do was dance in my own way, in order to feel heard, in order to connect. It very much takes us back to the initial purpose of dance. Without all the athletics and acrobatics, you are left with freedom; freedom to translate the effect of the world and the effect of your emotions on you, into movement, the highest form of music. I recently connected with Simon Jarrett author of *Those They Called Idiots* and editor of *Community Living Magazine* and his work in the field of dance and learning disabilities is incredibly inspirational to me.

When they heard through a friend, about the dance sessions I was doing with people with learning disabilities, Northern Ballet got in touch and asked me to teach at their wheelchair ballet class for their In Motion course in the summer of 2022 as their artist in residence.

To get an actual job with Northern Ballet is yet another dream come true. I have watched this dance company ever since I was child. I revered those dancers and to now think I am to be a part of the same company, a part of their history and legacy, is just overwhelming.

People have referred to me as inspirational, but I would reject that word mainly because it puts too much pressure on me and suggests I have no flaws. I do. Plenty of them. I used to be a perfectionist, before and after my injury. I was always trying to be enough for everybody else. The model employee, the model sister, the model daughter, even the model CES patient. But it was exhausting because of course, I could never be that image of perfection I had in my mind.

These days I'm simply trying to be enough for myself.

I recently wrote an activity book for people with learning disabilities, which contains little reminders to be kind to yourself, because I've learnt that being kind to myself changed everything for me. I strive against perfectionism now. And that was something, without realising the parallel back then, I always loved in my hero Margot Fonteyn, who eschewed the polish, for the passion. She found perfection in imperfection. And that's what I like to do these days. So, I'll take the compliment, but I don't see myself as *inspiring*. Take from my story what you will. If there were things in it you liked, that inspired you, then go be inspiring yourself!

I will now be sharing that message through the charity Bringing Us Together along with my good friend Nadia Clarke, who is also a disability advocate. She has cerebral palsy and together we are trying to encourage our community to be kinder to itself. We are huge proponents of the social model of disability, meaning that the only way we are *dis*-abled is because the world isn't accessible enough... yet.

I am an avid watcher of *Strictly* these days. It does such a wonderful job of bringing people together, of promoting positivity and making the marginalized become the mainstream. Whether it is same sex couples, amputees, older people or even the deaf, everyone is celebrated and can be seen to reach great heights of attainment. I have been on the receiving end of hate crime and now I work with organizations to help eradicate it by focusing on inclusion and normalizing diversity in that *Strictly* style, so that one day hopefully there won't be that fear of the unknown attached to diversity that causes people to react so negatively when they see someone who doesn't look or even move like them.

For a long time, I thought dancing and disability excluded one another. Now I know that that isn't the case at all. Far from it.

My seventy-six-year-old mum joins in with the dance classes I take these days and it always makes me smile. It brings my dad's words flooding back to me on that day we ate ice cream looking up at Big Ben.

'You came along so your mum would always have someone to dance with.'

He was absolutely right.

To this day we still dance together.

In ways we never dreamed of.

I would like to thank Mr Timothy my spinal consultant for the proactive approach he took to my care that has enabled me to have this beautiful life with my nephews, nieces, Godchildren, Mum and, not forgetting, my cats.

DUNCAN'S STORY

I Can
... and so can you.

Blue were riding high.

Our first album (2001's *All Rise*) had been certified four times platinum in the UK, spending sixty-three weeks in the Top 75. We'd had four singles from it in the top ten, two of those had gone to number one, and now our second album *One Love*, on which we got to work with none other than the bone fide superstar Elton John, entered the charts at number one, also going platinum four times over.

Our fan base was huge and still growing fast. We were now able to fill massive venues so, our first ever arena tour was booked, and rehearsals were underway. It was intense. While the band always had a breezy cool image with effortlessly slick performances, it took hours and hours of hard work behind the scenes to nail those routines.

It was during those rehearsals that I first started getting trouble with my back. It was more than a twinge; it was really, *really,* painful and it was going down my leg too. So, I went to my doctor and got an MRI scan, which revealed that one of the discs in my spine was bulging and rubbing on my sciatic nerve. I told him I was in rehearsals for the biggest tour of my career so far and I needed something to make sure this condition didn't ruin it for me and the rest of the band. He said a nerve root block epidural would do the trick, one simple injection – and it worked. It was amazing. That was in 2002 and for the next ten years I didn't have any pain or any problems with my back. Job done.

Or so I thought.

In 2011, after being apart since 2005, Blue reformed and smashed it at The Eurovision Song Contest with a song I co-wrote called *I Can*. We came in a very respectable 11th place (or 5^{th,} if the viewing public had had their way, according to the official voting figures). The song was an uplifting song, with a rousing lyric all about getting back up again after a loss or a fall, something which I was going to have to do big time with regards to my health soon enough.

The following year we recorded a comeback album and were all pleased to see that demand for the band was still high. That would mean plenty of shows and plenty of hard work again.

But that was OK. I wasn't afraid of hard work.

I'd been working full-time since the age of sixteen. My mum was a single parent, so money was a bit tight growing up. She went out to work all hours as a nurse and was often doing night shifts, which meant, as a kid, I was looked after by my grandparents for a lot of the time.

We lived an army base life. My grandfather was a colonel in the Royal Signals and during the war my grandmother was in the RAF. By the time I came along, Grandad had retired from the army and was working as a music teacher in a private school. I was lucky enough to attend that school until I was nine, but then the fees became too expensive, and I had to go to a good old comprehensive instead.

My grandmother hated any loud music in the house, so I had to listen to the Top 40 secretly on headphones; the only thing allowed was the piano. Every night my grandad would play, and I would sit next to him watching what he was doing and picking up how to play in the process. Every weekend he would play piano at the garrison church, and I loved going along with him. The guards at the gate would salute my colonel granddad as we drove through. I thought that was so cool. Perhaps that was one of the things that sparked my love affair with fame – that and going to Butlins where my mum took me on holiday.

I dreamed of being a Redcoat and performing for a living. Unlike my grandparents, Mum would have no qualms about pumping out classic 70s and 80s pop from the radio when we were together, and we would dance around the house as I dreamed of being a singer.

Mum and I have always been super close. She would always encourage me to follow my dreams and go for what I wanted. I loved acting and I would be in every school play, every drama group production and I always managed to bag the lead roles and make a name for myself in the small pond of school life before trying to do the same out in the big wide world of professional showbiz.

All of us boys in Blue had been through some ups and some downs separately and as a band over the decade since 2002. We had gone from nobodies to somebodies. We'd gone from topping the charts to splitting up. We'd gone from living a champagne lifestyle to bankruptcy. So, when in 2012 we had the opportunity to hit the road again, I wasn't about to let a bit of hard graft get in the way.

But what *did* get in the way were my back problems again when the pain returned with a vengeance.

So, I popped off to the doctors and got another epidural and everything was fine for another few years until 2015 when I was so excited to land the role of Tick in the stage musical version of *Priscilla, Queen of the Desert.* Rehearsals for this were unlike anything I had done before with Blue, mainly because I had to wear enormously high heels for most of it. And that took its toll on my problematic back.

Ten days away from opening night I could barely walk, the pain in my back was so intense. So back to the doctor I went, and another MRI showed that the disc bulge was getting worse and the best thing to do, I was told, would be to have an operation where they would shave the bit of the disc away that was causing the pain.

'That's just not a possibility,' I said to the doctor. 'My new show opens in just over a week. How about another of those injections? They worked so well before.'

The doctor explained that the injections were only a quick fix. They weren't really dealing with the root of the problem, and they couldn't help in the long run. But what could I do? I had a job to do, and I was the 'name' that was going to get bums on seats for the tour. I didn't want to let the cast and crew down. And I was also very concerned about the public perception of me – a natural side effect of being in a high-profile pop band for so many years. I was worried that people would think I couldn't handle the role of Tick after all, and that I was pretending to be off sick for six weeks to delay having to perform. I didn't feel I had a choice. I had to do the tour.

I had the epidural and for the first six months of the tour everything was fine. But the effect of the injection wore off much quicker this time, and the pain started to return yet again. With my work schedule ruling surgery out as far as I was concerned, my doctor suggested I try other things to manage the pain, like acupuncture and massage. Travelling to a different city every week, I would also have physio before and after the show. But one Monday morning I woke up in Bristol, where we were just about to open at the Hippodrome, and I couldn't get out of bed. I called my doctor in a panic. I told him I needed the epidural again. And fast.

My doctor was up to his elbows performing another operation, so he told me, 'Get yourself to Charing Cross hospital and I'll arrange for someone to give you the injection there.'

Somehow, I made it onto a train, but I was in such agony that the only way I could cope with the journey was to lie on the floor of the carriage. People had to step over me as they moved through the train, but there was nothing else I could do. I had never experienced agony like it before, or since. I staggered off the train and into a black cab, which I also lay on the floor of, all the way to Charing Cross hospital, where I was put straight on a gurney and wheeled inside.

The anaesthetist there told me a scan wasn't necessary as I had had one just a few months before, so he gave me the epidural I was clucking for and sent me home, telling me the pain would ease off within twenty-four hours.

I chose not to go home and be alone. There was something about the pain that was so unusual I knew it wasn't right. Luckily, my great friend Tara Palmer-Tomkinson lived on Earls Court Road, just around the corner from the hospital, so I called her up and asked if I could stay with her for the night.

She came straight round and brought me to her place, where I lay on the kitchen floor.

'This isn't right,' I repeated. 'The pain usually wears off by now after an injection.'

'You know what you need, darling,' she said in true Tara style. 'A shot of vodka. That will sort you out. Always works for me.'

She went to the fridge and poured me shot after shot until the pain turned to giggles. Tara was such a great friend and she stayed by my side for hours trying to keep my spirits up. However, in the night I could feel my left leg going numb, so I frantically messaged my doctor telling him this, to which he replied, 'Don't worry, it's just the strength of the epidural. Give it a bit more time and everything will be fine.'

Tara gave me a sleeping pill to compliment the vodka and I managed to knock myself out until eight in the morning when I woke up dying for a wee. But I couldn't go. No matter how hard and how often I tried, nothing would come out.

This was very weird. My left leg was completely numb and now I'd lost the ability to pee. Were the two things connected?

I called a friend of mine, who happened to be a doctor, and told him my symptoms. He told me that, if I could get myself down to the scanning centre in Harley Street, he could book me in at 9AM that same day for an MRI.

MRIs can last for anything from thirty minutes to an hour and a half, but I had been in the machine for about ten minutes when the radiologist stopped the scan and came into the room telling me the disc in my spine had completely dislodged and torn allowing the jelly inside it to ooze onto the sciatic nerve, which was beginning to kill it off.

'You need emergency surgery,' he said. 'Now!'

Wide-eyed with panic, I was taken back to the Charing Cross hospital, but the surgeon who I had been seeing about my back over the years, was not able to do the operation on me. He was in the middle of a nine-hour surgery to remove a tumour from someone's brain but managed to take time out for a minute to explain that they were trying to find another surgeon who could do it. I would have been happy to wait for him, but he told me that if the surgery wasn't done soon, I would go into what's known as Cauda Equina Syndrome.

I had never heard of this condition, but it was clear that this was very serious.

He looked at his watch and said, 'We're probably about thirty-two hours in since these particular symptoms manifested.'

I nodded.

'After forty hours,' he said, 'there could be irreparable damage to your mobility, bladder and bowels, and sexual function. You can't afford to wait for me.'

So, as they searched for another surgeon qualified to do such a risky operation, I lay there as if there were a timebomb under my bed. To say I was nervous was an understatement. My Mum arrived at my bedside, and we helplessly watched the hands turn on the clock, preparing for the worst if another doctor wasn't found in time – the worst being that I might never walk again. Both Mum and I were scared beyond belief.

When the thirty-eighth hour came, a registrar appeared. He was Italian and spoke little English bless him, but he was able to tell me, quite honestly, that he had never actually done the operation I needed before. However, he had been trained to do it, he explained, and in the absence of anyone else, he was, frankly, my last resort.

'Have faith in me,' he said reassuringly.

I was not reassured, but what else could I do?

I went under.

When I came round, I was told that the operation had been a success. The sciatic nerve had been freed from the obstruction and I was going to be fine.

This was more than good news and after a couple of days of recovery in hospital I was allowed to go home.

But then I started getting these terrible headaches, and not ones that could be sorted out with a couple of Paracetamol. Every time I stood up, I felt as if my head was about to explode but if I lay down the headache went away. It was yet another bizarre sensation, and, yet again, one I had never experienced before.

I called the surgeon who explained that it could possibly be a cerebrospinal fluid leak from the trauma of the surgery and asked me to come to hospital where I had to lay prone on a bed for three days. If there was a tear in the Dural sac, (the membranous sac that encases and protects the cauda equina nerves and the spinal cord within the bony structure of the vertebral column) then, during that time, it would repair itself as long as I stayed in the same position so it had time to heal. It was not only very boring laying there, but it was really unnerving having to be face downwards like that for three long days. However, at the end of it I was sent home, supposedly all healed.

Two weeks later, on a Saturday night, my Mum and I were at home watching *X-factor*. As we watched young Louisa Johnson smash yet another song out of the park with her effortless vocal power and range, I was distracted by this dampness under my bottom. I stood up and saw the chair was wet. I reached down and my trousers were wet too.

'What's going on?' I said, 'Mum, have a look at my scar, would you?'

She could see this clear liquid pouring from the scar on my back, so we quickly called the surgeon and told him what was happening. His response didn't exactly help me relax.

'Shit' he said. 'Right, lay on the floor face down! I'm calling an ambulance now. Don't touch the area around the scar with dirty hands; keep it clean! Use alcohol wipes if you have them. If that fluid gets any infection in it, there's a huge risk you will get meningitis.'

After a tense wait, for both me and my Mum, the ambulance arrived and I was heading back to Charing Cross where the surgeon greeted me with the words, 'I'm going to operate on you tonight. We must find the source of the leak and stop it right away.'

When I came round from this second operation, my surgeon told me that he hadn't been able to find the leak, so instead he sprayed the entire area with a kind of surgical glue that should solve the problem wherever it was. He also said he found some more of the jelly that the registrar had missed, pressing on the sciatic nerve, but that had now been cleared away and the surgeon expected that I would have no more problems.

The pain and the headaches had finally disappeared, but for a couple of weeks after the surgery I had to be hooked up to a catheter because I still couldn't feel anything in my bladder. Every so often the catheter would be clamped to see if I could feel the build-up of urine in my bladder, and eventually I felt the need to go.

'That's a great sign,' the doctor smiled.

I'd never been so pleased to need a wee.

Unfortunately, the feeling in my left leg never returned. To this day, from my bum down to my knee and along the left side of my foot, I can't feel anything. This was really worrying at first. I couldn't run anymore, and I would walk with a pronounced limp as my leg had no power in it to propel me forward. This was upsetting enough in my day-to-day life, but as a performer it was unthinkable. I always used to imagine I would do quite well if I ever got asked to do *Strictly Come Dancing*, but now I don't think I'd get very far. I joke about it, but it does sadden me.

Two weeks after the second operation, I was due to begin working up in Liverpool on *Hollyoaks* playing the role of Ryan Knight. I was still recovering and doped up to my eyeballs on tramadol, but there was no way I could jeopardize the two-year contract they had offered me.

In hindsight I wished I had taken more time off, rested and concentrated on rehabilitation. But soap operas wait for no man! And if I didn't start now my character would have been written out before he even appeared. It was a toss-up: a few more weeks rest or two years of high-profile work guaranteed. Once again it was a no brainer for me. I had to suck it up and get on with it.

My Mum moved up to Liverpool with me for the first couple of months of the job. She was a godsend, and as a nurse she came into her own at this time for me. I couldn't have done it without her. She'd been by my side since that first operation and now, bless her, she helped me get dressed and helped me tie my laces because I was still in loads of pain.

The physical pain was bad enough, but mentally it was a strain too. There were days when I just wanted to quit. I didn't want to go into work. I didn't want to pick up a script and try to learn all these lines, because they weren't going into my tramadol-addled brain properly. I couldn't concentrate or focus, and I felt like crying. I felt like giving up. I had to dig deep and with help from my mum I kept going and got through it. I'm so grateful to my mum for being there for me through thick and thin. And I'm proud of myself, for making it through. Never before had the lyrics of our Eurovision song *I Can* meant so much. I had to get back up again.

I was still limping and using a walking stick, but my character Ryan Knight didn't. So, all my scenes in

Hollyoaks had to be shot from the waist up, or I'd be propping up the bar in the pub or leaning against the kitchen counter; always positioned so I never had to walk anywhere on camera.

The filming schedule was a busy one and I was very happy to be working, but it left little time for me to concentrate on getting the physio I needed to improve my walking. I had health insurance which meant I could have private health care ever since my back problems started, but the trouble with going private is, often after a surgery, you are not offered any follow up appointments or advice for the future. As a private patient, you have to initiate this stuff yourself, which the NHS would often do for you as a matter of course, and when you do request it, it comes at a cost. My medical insurance bills were enormous after my operations and, contrary to what you might think, soap stars don't get paid a lot.

All these factors conspired against me, so that I didn't get enough aftercare in the weeks and months beyond my surgery. That's why, about a year into the show, I started to get bad pins and needles in my right hand. A scan showed I now had a disc bulge in my neck because my spine was out of alignment due to the uneven way I had been walking since the operations.

It seemed like these problems would never end.

However, my doctor referred me to a podiatrist, who assessed me and had some orthotics made for me. Wearing them in my shoes levelled out my uneven gait and miraculously the neck problems vanished.

Having talked about the cons of private care, I must mention the pros, and add that the speed with which you can get seen if you go private is crucial when it comes to something like Cauda Equina Syndrome. I know first-hand how time is the critical factor when getting successful treatment for CES. You cannot afford to wait until next week, you cannot afford to wait hours; people need to know the warning signs and they need to insist on getting help. You know your own body. You know when something is not right. And if the first doctor you see doesn't give you a satisfactory response, go and get a second opinion, as I did. Without claiming on my health insurance, I paid directly for the scan which first revealed that I was going into Cauda Equina Syndrome, and it was the best hundred and fifty quid I ever spent. Sure, that's not a small amount of money, but what price can you put on your ability to walk and to have a functioning bladder and bowels for the rest of your life?

I was so sad when I had to quit *Priscilla, Queen of the Desert* because of my first operation. It was such a great role in a fabulous show, and I doubted if I'd ever have an opportunity to do anything like it again. But then in 2018 I landed my dream role: the part of Frank N. Furter in *The Rocky Horror Show*. The big challenge with this part, however, was that like Tick, Frank N. Furter wears outrageously fabulous heels.

It was probably an unusual day for my doctors when I turned up for scans and assessments mainly to establish whether I could wear stilettoes for months on end, but they gave me the all-clear, providing Frank N. Furter wore orthotics in his high heels, and as long as I took good care of myself. And so, taking on the doctor's advice, the dream job was mine.

I was so happy to be back on stage performing every night and I was also thankful every day that I had not ended up in a wheelchair and catheterized for the rest of my life, as many people with Cauda Equina Syndrome unfortunately are.

As we go into 2022, I am rehearsing for my latest musical role in *War of the Worlds*. I'm not in heels this time, but it's still a wonderful job. And one day I'd love to get another crack at *Priscilla, Queen of the Desert* – although I might be more suitable for the role of the old dame Bernadette by then. Nevertheless, that would be amazing. Just to have the opportunity to still be working and performing is a gift I don't take for granted anymore.

I took the quick fix when I first had big problems with my back during *Priscilla, Queen of the Desert*. I should have taken a more, long term view and chosen the microdiscectomy over the epidural. If I had done that and taken just six weeks out of *Priscilla*, I might have never gone into Cauda Equina Syndrome and could have avoided the emergency surgery. Also, I might not have been left with the problems with my leg that I have now.

When Cauda Equina Syndrome happened to me, suddenly I found myself questioning my own mortality in a way I'd never thought about before. I had always been gym fit and healthy, but CES was a wakeup call for me. I realised I had to be kinder to myself and look after my body better. Banging out a load of weights in the gym is not looking after yourself if you have back issues. Instead, strengthening your core muscles is an essential focus for fitness and something which I take a lot more seriously these days, as I do my food choices and my vices. Abusing your body and pushing yourself too far are just not options if you want to stay strong.

I was on *Loose Women* once talking about my condition and after that a lot of people and charities reached out to me to let me know that I was not alone. That was a real comfort to me. Kind of like when I told the world I was gay.

When I came out, I had such a wonderful response from people telling me how it helped them take courage and share their truth too. My experience with Cauda Equina Syndrome is a story which is just as important to share. Knowing the signs that you may be going into CES is so important. And knowing that it is your right to insist on the appropriate help from your doctors can literally change the rest of your life with such a time sensitive issue.

That's why I became an Ambassador for the Cauda Equina Champions Charity. I would be over the moon if me talking about the condition with the large platform I have, saves even one person from going into CES and avoids them having to use a wheelchair for the rest of their life, or debilitating bladder and bowel issues and loss of sexual function, which I was lucky enough to avoid. And if we can save a lot more than one, then all the better.

When you suffer with a condition like CES, your confidence is knocked. I know, because mine was. Suddenly I became aware of how fragile I felt physically too. Things I always thought I'd do, were no longer possible. I was no longer the invincible person I thought I was. I was in my late thirties when it happened to me, and I had a lot of plans for my future. I'd had a career which allowed me to do all sorts of amazing things and I couldn't imagine that ever changing. But of course, life is what happens to you while you're busy making other plans, as someone once wisely said. And it's at times like these, when you feel at your most vulnerable, that you need to know you are not alone. There are many people going through the same thing, far too many in fact. It's terrifying, yes, but we need to look at all the things we can do, not the things we can't. And if you reach out to organizations like the Cauda Equina Champions Charity you will find support and, through sharing stories or through simply talking through your fears, you'll find the strength to go on, I promise. If *I can*, then so can you.

I want to say a big shout out to the nursing staff at The Charing Cross hospital, who were so wonderful during my time there. These nurses come from all corners of the globe to grace our National Health Service with their dedication and compassion. Thank you all for making such a lovely fuss of me!

OSCAR'S STORY

My family are a premier league team.

My name is Oscar.

I am ten years old. I live near Bolton with my Mum, Dad, our two daft dogs Otis and Nellie, and my two brothers Charlie and Freddie. Charlie is fifteen and Freddie is nine. There is only about thirteen months age difference between Freddie and me. We are close in age and close as brothers. We even share a bedroom. Every night when we go to bed, we stay awake chatting until Dad comes in and tells us we should be asleep.

In school, all three of us love maths and sports. I love maths because it's not confusing with loads of opinions. In maths the answer is either right or wrong. There's no in between. That makes a lot of sense.

I love playing football most of all. I play it during school playtime, after school and at the weekends. I play for a local team. I'm football mad, just like my dad. We're both fans of Manchester United. My dad took me to see my first ever match at Old Trafford last year, at the start of the season in 2021. It was amazing.

Dad played football when he was a kid too. And rugby. But when he was in his twenties, he got this blood condition called Factor V Leiden which meant he could sometimes get blood clots in his legs, so he had to give up playing things like rugby and football. I'd be gutted if that was me. I think he was gutted too, but he always says to us, 'Get out of your comfort zone! You can do more than you think you can.' And that's why he didn't give up on sports. He just started running instead. He would go out most evenings after work training, going further and further each

102

time until he even did a half marathon. He said running is hard at first. Whoever you are. It's not something you really enjoy. You have to force yourself to get out there and do it, but then if you stick at it, you start to get addicted in a good way. A bit like getting up for school every day.

When COVID19 came along and everyone had to stay at home, it was a bit boring because I couldn't go to school or play football anymore. All the hairdressers were closed too so I couldn't get my hair cut. My mum and dad would have made a right mess of it if I'd let them have a go, so I just started to grow it. My hair always used to be quite short, so it was weird having longer hair at first. But my nanna told me that she thought it was lovely. Then she had this idea. I could raise money for charity, getting sponsored to grow my hair and then, if I grew it long enough, when the time came to cut it, I could donate the hair to the Little Princess Trust, which makes wigs for kids who've lost their hair because of cancer treatment. I thought this was a great idea. I like helping people.

My parents always say that I'm a happy kid. That's a bit embarrassing, but I know what they mean. I like to have a laugh and a joke. I don't want to think about bad stuff. I want everyone to be happy. So, I try to be positive. We were in a car crash a few years ago which really scared me. Every time I'm in a car now I am quite nervous, but I try not show it. I don't want my family to worry about me.

When lockdown was over and we could go back to school, my hair wasn't long enough to donate to the Little Princess Trust. It had to be twelve inches long or more. So, I had to keep growing it for a few more months.

Some of the kids at school were surprised to see me with such long hair. And I got a lot of stick from some of them. I had to put my hair in a ponytail when I was at school, so they started calling me a girl and stuff like that.

That was upsetting so I went home one day and said to my dad, 'Would it be all right if I cut my hair before it's ready for the charity? Would you be disappointed?'

My dad said, 'If you want to get it cut, that's your choice. No one's going to force you to cut it. But look how far you've come? Do you want to give up now?'

It was like he was talking about doing a marathon – he'd just signed up to do the Edinburgh Marathon next year. And in a way I felt like I was a doing a marathon too. And I was quite close to the finish line. If I cut my hair now none of the kids with cancer would be able to use it. So, I decided to stick with it, even though when I went into public toilets some blokes would tell me I was in the wrong one. I wasn't sure if they were mistaking me for a girl or just being horrible.

One Friday night in November 2021, Mum and Dad were going to IKEA shopping. Me and my brothers hate doing that, so we went to stay with Nanna instead. Dad reckons she spoils us. We have a great time there. We go out to the park, and we eat loads of sweets.

When we got home, Dad was moaning all weekend about having a sore back – he had hurt it bending down to pick something up in IKEA. On Monday morning he didn't get up for work like he usually does. Mum said his back was still playing up, but when I got home from school on Tuesday, Mum told me Dad was in hospital and he had to stay there overnight.

I cried because I was worried about him and because I didn't understand what was wrong. Mum said she didn't really know what was wrong either. No one seemed to know. But it was something to do with his back. He needed to have some tests done and a scan in the morning and that would help find out what was wrong.

It wasn't easy sleeping that night and I couldn't wait to get home the next day after school to see Dad.

But he didn't come home.

Mum said he was still in hospital, and he needed to have an operation on his back. She tried to make it sound like it was nothing to worry about, but I could see she was scared. I didn't get it. He only had a sore back the other day and now he was having surgery. I was really upset. I asked Mum when we would see Dad again. She said, 'Soon. Soon.' When adults say that it means they don't have a clue.

It was nearly a week later when Mum said we could go to see Dad. That week had felt like months, but at least now things were getting back to normal.

Then, the day before the visit, someone in the hospital ward Dad was on got COVID and all visits were cancelled. Dad was not allowed to see anyone at all. Everyone on the ward was separated. He was put in a room on his own for the next ten days.

Mum told us that Dad had this thing called Cauda Equina Syndrome. It was something to do with his spine. It meant he was having trouble walking now and going to the toilet properly. She said that when he got home, he wouldn't be able to do everything that he did before, and he would need a lot of help from us.

That was OK, I thought. I like helping people. I said to Mum, 'That's alright, coz we're a team. Like Man U. We all help each other.'

But it was so weird. I tried to imagine what he would look like when I saw him. I wondered if he would look different. I wondered if he would look the same. I wondered what he would be able to do and what he wouldn't be able to do. At school I did my best and concentrated hard on my lessons, but when I got outside at breaktime I would just zone-out thinking about all this stuff. This Cauda Equina thing didn't make sense. It wasn't straightforward like maths. But I knew it wasn't right. I missed my dad so much.

I was nervous, but really excited to see Dad when the ten days quarantine was up, but the day before we were going to see him, the hospital changed the rules and Dad had to isolate for another four or five days. It must have been really hard for him, not being at home with us. It was really doing my head in too, all this waiting. I didn't want to talk to people much, and little things made me upset.

Mum had to go to work as usual, but without Dad at home me and my brothers had to spend a lot of time at my grandparents' house. Whenever we went home again, I used to hang around Mum a lot. I suppose I was worried she was going to disappear too.

After a couple of weeks, we were allowed to go and see Dad in the garden of the hospital. *Finally!* We all had lunch together. Dad was in a wheelchair which was shocking. I mean, old people and disabled people use wheelchairs, not my dad. But I made sure I had a joke and a laugh with him to make him feel better. The thing was, I didn't know if I would hurt him if I touched him.

'Are we allowed to give you a hug?' I asked.

Luckily the answer was yes. But I was very careful anyway.

It was so good to see Dad, but we had to wait another week until he was ready to come home. So, I just told myself that he would be better soon. We'd be back down the Astroturf playing football again in no time.

Dad came home just before Christmas. He was getting about using crutches and he still had the wheelchair if we went out longer distances. It was a weird Christmas because we couldn't do all the things we usually do then.

Every year we'd go to see the pantomime at the theatre in Bolton, but this year we couldn't. We also couldn't go on massive walks like we used to with Otis and Nellie.

But Dad kept telling us we had nothing to worry about. 'It's not like I have a terminal illness,' he'd say.

We all helped him as much as we could. I asked him all the time if he needed anything. Sometimes he needed me to pick something up for him. Sometimes I would bring him stuff. Mum would help him get dressed and help him with his physio exercises.

When the physiotherapist came to see my dad, Dad said to him, 'Push me!'

He didn't mean push him over. He meant, 'Push me to go further than even I think I can go.'

Dad said he needed to treat his recovery like a long-distance race. He said he needed to look back after every session every day and say, 'I went a little further today than I did yesterday.' He's very strong from all his years being sporty and active, and that helped him a lot after Cauda Equina, but he told me it's the mental strength that gets you across the finish line of a marathon more than the physical. And he needed to treat his recovery like a marathon. He needed to see that he could improve day by day, week by week.

And he did.

He would never sit around for long. He made sure he kept moving. And four months after the operation he can now walk a little way all by himself. Mostly he gets around on crutches to help him balance because his feet are still numb and don't work properly. He still needs the wheelchair, for long distances but he's definitely getting better.

Before Cauda Equina, Dad used to be at work a lot. Sometimes six days a week, until six o'clock at night. He was a scaffolder. Now he's at home a lot, and I like that. I get to see him much more. He takes us to school when Mum's out at work.

But I am sad that we can't go down the park and play footie together anymore. I thought we would eventually get to do that, but there might be some things that Dad just can't do like he used to anymore.

By January 2022 my hair was finally long enough to cut for the charity. It had been just over two years since I last had it cut. I couldn't wait to get it off.

Mum's auntie has a hair salon. That was the place that I had my first ever hair cut when I was little and that was the place where we were going to cut my hair for the Little Princess Trust.

I also knew now who I was going to donate all the money I'd raised through people sponsoring me to.

At first, I'd thought about a charity which helps people who've had stillborn babies because Mum's sister had gone through that a few years before. But then, since Dad got Cauda Equina he'd been in touch with this charity called The Cauda Equina Champions Charity. I had seen how they had given my dad loads of help and support. He had been able to talk to other people with the same condition and people who had faced the same problems he had. They found a therapist for him and Mum to help them with the big changes they were going through. They even got us t-shirts made for my sponsored hair growing. They had been so brilliant and helped my dad so much, I knew the right thing to do was to help them back.

A journalist came to our house and did a story for the local newspaper and then we went to the salon for the big day. Loads of friends and family came too. Also, Claire from the Cauda Equina Champions Charity came, and it was brilliant to be able to give her £2000 for her charity and give all my hair to the Little Princess Trust. It was so weird to have short hair again, but I was glad I wouldn't be getting anymore stick.

Dad gets a little bit better every day, which is brilliant. Some things will never get back to the way they were, but Dad sees it as an opportunity. For example, he thinks he won't be able to do scaffolding ever again, but he often thought about going back to college and trying something new. He just never got round to it. Now, it looks like he might have the chance to.

Even the smallest things can be a challenge for him, but he always keeps going. He says it's hard to explain, but he tells me long distance running and recovery from Cauda Equina Syndrome are similar. You should force yourself to get out there and do it at first, but then, if you stick at it, you see yourself going further than you did last time and then one day you realise you can do it, you can do what you never thought possible.

Get out of your comfort zone! You can do more than you think you can.

That was his motto before his accident.

And it still is today.

And I think that's pretty cool!

A message from Oscar's dad, Chris:

I would like to say a special thank you to my spinal nurses Clare Bluer and Kelly Jackson at Salford Royal Hospital. Without them I wouldn't have had the help and knowledge that I needed before being discharged.

Also, I owe a massive thank you to my neuro-physiotherapist Dave Berry, who has pushed me (not over) every time I see him, and he has helped my physical development so much more than I could have hoped for so far. I've got a long journey ahead of me, but I'm sure he'll take me as far as he can along that road.

Finally, I want to thank my family, especially my wife Katy. She helped me every day with my physio, helped me get dressed and I don't think I would be where I am in my recovery now without her. She has been my absolute rock, so understanding. A godsend, mentally and physically.

STEVEN'S STORY

You can't drive a chair.

Cars. I can't get enough of them. Cars, cars, cars, cars, cars.

But I'm not the kind of bloke who tinkers under the bonnet all day. I'm not a mechanic in any way. I'm useless at that. I just love driving. I like moving at high speeds. I love sports cars, high performance cars. That's why when an opportunity came up to become a traffic policeman, I jumped at it.

I'd been in the force since I was eighteen. My dad was a police officer, and I don't remember ever wanting to be anything else as I grew up in Blackpool, Lancashire. But when I signed up, the only area recruiting at that time in the late eighties was the Met in London, so I upped sticks and moved to the Big Smoke.

I was stationed in central London so spent a lot of time on the job dealing with tourists, which made it a lot of fun, on the whole. But the cost of living was a lot higher than I was used to up North, so after five years of expensive living, and to be closer to home, I found a job with the Greater Manchester Police.

That was when I got my chance to work as a traffic officer on motorways. The opportunity to be around, and in, cars all day was just too good to be true for this petrol head. But of course, it wasn't all fun by any means. Being a traffic officer meant dealing with accidents. A lot of the accidents were horrific and those involving children, some of whom died in my arms, stay with you forever. There's also a lot of high-speed chases, people ramming into you, bumps and scrapes and physical altercations. So, I got quite a few back injuries from all this, which resulted in a lot of twinges and pain over the years.

In 2002 my third son was born prematurely and had to be kept at hospital in an incubator for five or six weeks. Not long after we finally got him home from hospital, I had to be rushed into hospital.

I had been having sciatica for a while with a painful back ache and then one day I found I couldn't walk at all. It turned out one of my discs had prolapsed and so when I got to hospital they gave me a discectomy, where the part of the disc, which is pressing on the spinal cord and causing the pain, is removed.

That sorted me out in terms of the acute pain, but there was always a lot of intermittent pain and twinges after that and so five years later in 2007 I had to be medically retired from the force because of the ongoing issues with my back. I had been with the force for twenty years by then. They had offered me a desk job, but my response was:

'You can't drive a chair, can you?'

I couldn't imagine being sat behind a desk all day when all I wanted to be do was be out there on the motorways driving and making a difference to the safety of those on the roads. That's what I was trained to do. And I loved it. Driving was everything to me. I'd done every single driving course you could possibly do to develop myself in this branch of policing: high speed driving, VIP driving. protection driving, 4x4 driving, HGV driving, you name it, I'd done it. So, when I left the police, I really missed the driving part more than anything.

I didn't have any major issues with my back again until 2010. It was the week before Christmas, and I was out looking for a nice present for my wife. I was chuffed when I found what I was looking for, but as I was walking back to the car, I was suddenly aware that I'd wet myself. It was not only the strangest thing, but embarrassing too. I was right in the middle of the bustling town at one of the busiest times of the year.

'What is going on?' I thought to myself as I hurried back to safety of my beloved car.

I went home and told my wife, and she encouraged me to call the G.P. He responded very quickly and told me to come in and see him immediately. After giving me an assessment, he said it was clear to him that I had this thing he called Cauda Equina Syndrome. It was a rare condition, he said, and I was only the second person he had ever seen with it. He called an ambulance right away and they took me to Blackpool Victoria Hospital.

Being the Friday before Christmas, the hospital was rammed with festive casualties, and I got swallowed up in the crowd. I arrived at noon, and it wasn't until the early hours of the following morning, after I'd been sitting there uncomfortably for fifteen hours, that some bright spark realised this hospital wasn't the right one for someone in my condition who needed neurosurgery, so I was shipped over to Preston and put on a ward there, where I waited for a scan…

…for FOUR DAYS.

Apparently, they were so backed up that that was the quickest I could get seen.

After looking at my MRI a clinical nurse specialist confirmed I had Cauda Equina Syndrome, but the neurosurgeon assigned to me disagreed. Many other people involved in my care in that hospital spoke of Cauda Equina as being the clear cause of my problems, but eventually, after much humming and hawing on the neurosurgeon's part, he went ahead and carried out the procedure that he was convinced I needed: an L5-S1 discectomy – the same

113

thing that I had back in 2002 and not the kind of surgery required if you have Cauda Equina Syndrome.

And then, after a few days recovering in hospital, on Christmas Eve I was told to go home. No advice other than, 'Take it easy and come back and see us in three months' time!'

So off I hobbled.

As you can imagine, our family Christmas was the worst Christmas ever for me. I was in too much pain to enjoy it. I could barely walk, and I was still having incontinence issues, so after New Year I called up the hospital and told them the situation.

'You *should* be fine,' they told me. 'Just give it a little more time!'

I gave it a little more time, but nothing was changing. It was unbearable so I went into the hospital to show them how difficult it was for me to walk.

They gave me a pair of crutches, telling me to come back in a few months.

I couldn't – and still cannot – walk without crutches, so I was supplied with a wheelchair, but I could never bring myself to use it. The moment I resorted to using a wheelchair was, in my mind, the moment I gave up. Yes, I know I'm a stubborn idiot, but there was something too final about the wheelchair. Something which suggested there was no way back from it; that I would just deteriorate even more if I sat in a chair every day. Just like when they offered me a desk job in the police force.

You can't drive a chair!

But with hindsight my stubbornness gave me more problems, not fewer. Now my right leg has started to suffer, I have issues with my hips and osteoarthritis in my shoulders because of using the crutches so much. And yet still I feel I would not be the person I am, doing everything

I do, if I used a wheelchair. Clearly for others it works, but it's just not me.

I realised, there is at least one chair you can drive: a mobility scooter. So if I have to mooch around town now, I go in that. I feel like an old fart, but at least in Blackpool I blend in with the countless other retirees whizzing around on their coffin dodgems.

During those weeks and months after the New Year, feeling completely lost in limbo and not listened to, I fell into a deep depression. I didn't really know it at the time, I didn't think anything was wrong with my state of mind, I thought it was everyone else around me that was the problem. But my family knew differently. You see, I had always had a sharp sense of humour. I was able to laugh most things off, but now my loved ones saw me changing, becoming moody and snappy, to such an extent that my wife said:

'If you don't get yourself sorted you won't have a family left.'

That was enough of a slap in the face for me to pull my finger out, so I went to my G.P. and he referred me to a counsellor.

Getting counselling was the best thing I ever did.

Just talking through my fears and feeling listened to was crucial. Reflecting on my life and realising how much I had to live for was vital in recalibrating my thought patterns and bringing me out of the doldrums. It helped me take charge of my problems and be responsible for finding solutions, reframing everything in a more positive way.

I never looked back.

Using crutches was still a struggle so I went to see my G.P. again and thankfully, he was a breath of fresh air compared to the hospital. He referred me to all the people I needed to see. He got me into a physio programme and found me a neurologist, who confirmed I had Cauda Equina Syndrome, though the consultant who I was under at the hospital still refused to accept that diagnosis. Nevertheless, the neurologist taught me about self-catheterisation to help me with the ongoing bladder issues and found me help in the form of medication and injections to help with the sexual dysfunction that often comes with CES.

I was also referred to a pain management clinic who arranged for me to be fitted with a spinal cord stimulator, which was cutting edge technology at the time. It's a device which is implanted under the skin and attaches to the spine sending low levels of electricity directly into the spinal cord to relieve pain. The downside is that I need charge myself up like a mobile phone every day. I stick a pad over the battery that protrudes from under my skin in to keep the stimulator working and the pain at bay. It is extremely effective for relieving the pain in my back and upper leg, but the nerve damage in my lower left leg is so severe, that it cannot help there. Consequently, I feel severe pain in that lower leg every day, all day. I take medication to try and relieve the pain, but it's always there.

With my new positive outlook, thanks to counselling, I soon found that the best way to avoid wallowing in my own problems was to help other people with theirs. So, I started helping out at the Cauda Equina Champions Charity by meeting with other sufferers, helping neurosurgeons with case studies, and giving speeches to medical professionals on the condition. One such time we went along to a training conference for one hundred and fifty paramedics, none of whom had ever heard of CES, but who all by the end of my speech, rose to give me a standing ovation as well as plenty of high fives on the car park!

The more people I met with CES the more it sank in that CES affects everyone in different ways. I had managed to avoid any bowel issues with my CES. Other people have severe issues with bowels and bladder but have no issues walking. But most of us suffer with depression at some point on the journey.

One of the greatest tools in getting through this for me has been my sense of humour. That's something which I almost lost for a while there after the operation at Christmas 2012. Thankfully I got it back and I use it whenever I talk to other people about the condition to show them that it's not all doom and gloom, and there is a way out of the negative thoughts which inevitably descend on us after the trauma of Cauda Equina Syndrome.

With neurological pain, often just being aware of it can make the pain more prominent. Distracting yourself and keeping busy can often be the best pain relief. That's why I'm so occupied these days doing the things I love. Not only do I spend time helping as Trustee at Cauda Equina Champions Charity, but I also became Chair of the board of governors at a local primary school as well as commander of the Blackpool Police Cadet Unit. I still get involved with the police force by going up to headquarters and helping with role plays in the training of new recruits and I've even acquired a teacher training qualification so I can train teachers in the police cadets.

And I count my blessings every day that I can still drive a car. If I need to go anywhere, I'll always choose to drive there if I can. If I couldn't drive anymore, I really would feel a sense of loss greater than any other I've felt throughout this ordeal. Driving still gives me that thrill I need; it still fulfils my need for speed – within the legal limits, of course.

Many, many thanks to G.P. Dr Hanif of the North Shore Surgery in Blackpool for his quick recognition of my condition and for promptly sending me to hospital.

Also, to Mr Nick Park, neurosurgeon at Preston Royal Hospital for all his help and guidance.

They both made a real difference and for that I am eternally grateful.

GINETTE'S STORY

Hospital hoppers

Everything about my childhood was wonderfully normal.

I was born in 1974 and grew up in Hertfordshire on the outskirts of London. I was the middle child of three with two brothers and we were, and still are, a very loving and supportive family.

I worked hard in school and achieved good grades. I had to because I knew I wanted to go into medicine in some way or another. Really, deep down I had made up my mind about this in secondary school, although when it was time to leave school, I was torn between a job in medicine and working for an airline. My Mum knew it was my dream to be a nurse and she encouraged that, but my dad wanted me to be an air stewardess. He was always fascinated by airplanes, and I think he might've wished he'd done the job himself once upon a time. But perhaps the main motivation for nudging me into working for an airline was all the free flights he imagined we'd get.

When I left school in the late eighties flying still had a lot of glamour attached to it and Virgin Atlantic was a relatively new airline injecting another level of cool into the job of cabin crew. So, I did apply and got an interview, but I knew very quickly that it wasn't for me. They wanted me to walk differently, wear make-up that didn't suit me and dress in clothes I didn't like. It felt like a bad modelling job rather than being in the aviation industry.

I went to college instead to do an NVQ in healthcare studies and started work for the NHS in 1990 in Watford General Hospital's Outpatients department. It wasn't long before I had experience in many aspects of nursing, in many different settings: A&E, surgical and paediatric, to name but a few. I moved around several hospitals over the years, but I loved my time in Mount Vernon A&E the most. It was a small unit with a close-knit team, which was very supportive of each other, out in the countryside, so not packed with the array of people that often turn up to A&E in inner city hospitals for bizarre reasons. You weren't overrun with belligerent drunks at the weekend, and you didn't get the hospital hoppers.

During my time in London, I heard the term *hospital hopper* for the first time. I learnt that it was the name given to someone who would lay down in the road or at the bottom of a flight of stairs pretending to be the victim of a hit and run or a fall just because they wanted to get a fix of morphine from the hospital.

But we didn't have hospital hoppers in Mount Vernon. The people that came there were truly in need of help.

So, I was sad when the powers that be decided to close Mount Vernon A&E and I was transferred to Watford A&E, which was at the other end of the spectrum. It was huge and not a pleasant place to work. As the new girl I got left with all the shifts that no one else wanted to take and I very quickly knew it was time for a change.

That's when I started thinking about the ambulance service and in 1997, I started training with London Ambulance Service as an Emergency Medical Technician, which is the role you had to do at the time before you could move on to being a paramedic with the extra responsibilities that entailed, such duties as intubating or delivering IV drugs where necessary. I did six weeks training in the classroom before spending a year on the road, learning on the job, alongside a qualified paramedic and even did some shifts as an observer on HEMS the

London Air Ambulance. As my work was all London based now, I saw everything imaginable and plenty that was unimaginable too.

However, by 2003 the commute to London was starting to become too much for me and when my third child was born with health issues, it confirmed my feeling that I needed a change of location. I managed to get a transfer to Watford Ambulance Station, closer to home.

Family has always been so important to me. I have always had great support from my brothers and parents. We all live near each other and would do anything for each other. We've always been very close like that.

However, in my household the cracks were beginning to show.

My husband was often physically abusive to me, but when my eldest child, who was just seven years old then, called me at work to tell me her father had been hitting her and her siblings on a regular basis too, enough was enough. I chucked my husband out and divorced him faster than you can say domestic abuse.

My husband was a police officer, and for many years I took the abuse because I thought no one would believe my word against his, a man of the law. I put up with it, I could take it I told myself, never thinking for a moment he would hit the children. But the children had kept quiet about the abuse they were getting because they thought I loved my husband, and they didn't want to be the ones to break up what they thought was a happy relationship, not knowing that he had been hitting me for years. Luckily, they found the strength to tell me eventually.

With that bad marriage behind me I found myself falling for someone else. Grant was a paramedic who I worked with. We had met a few years earlier when we both worked with St John's Ambulance Service, which I had done to get a feel for the job before committing to my EMT training. Then, when I moved to Watford Ambulance Station, Grant became my supervisor. We married in 2007 and in the November of the following year we had a beautiful baby girl called Neve.

It wasn't an easy birth though. I went into labour prematurely, after three weeks of intermittent pains. My consultant was concerned about this. So, at thirty-five weeks, when I went into labour prematurely yet again, he ordered an emergency C-section. Partly because the baby was clearly in some distress, and partly due to me having had two previous C-sections, which meant it was not advisable for me to give birth to Neve naturally.

Despite this, I didn't want to be unconscious through the birth, so I was told I could have an epidural, numbing everything from the waist down so I could be awake during the procedure. I had had epidurals for the births of my three other children to help with the pain, so I was quite familiar with the process and, as a medical professional myself, I knew exactly how they worked.

But this one wasn't going well at all. The doctor had real issues getting the epidural into my spine – the pain I felt as he tried again and again attested to that. He told me it was probably because of the other epidurals I had had in the past, which may have left a lot of scar tissue to get through. I didn't have any cause to debate that at the time. I was far more worried about getting Neve safely into the world. When she was delivered, she spent twenty-four hours in special care for some antibiotic treatment, but otherwise, Neve was just fine.

For me, however, it was a different story.

After the epidural wore off, I noticed that I still didn't have any sensation in my bladder. I told the nurse this and they did a scan which showed I had 1000ml of urine in there.

'You must feel something with that much in there,' she said.

'I don't,' I said, sensing that something wasn't right. I knew from my own training that any more than 600ml would cause the need to go to the toilet.

'Don't worry,' I was told. 'You've just had a caesarean. And you've had two before this. Your body needs time to recover. Go home and take it easy!'

So, I took Neve home, but the next day when the midwife came to visit, I still had not urinated. She did a scan, which revealed I now had 2 litres of urine in my bladder. Clearly there was something very wrong, not least because it took me half an hour to hobble with my husband and the midwife supporting me to the toilet, a journey which usually took me twenty seconds. The midwife recognised this and called for an ambulance.

It was weird to be in the back of an ambulance and not up front in my role as EMT, but I took some comfort that I was enroute to Watford where I knew a lot of the staff.

At the hospital a catheter was used to drain the urine, but no one seemed to be sure what the cause had been. In the end they put it down to the possibility that a nerve may have been nicked during the surgery, but once again, they said everything would be fine… in time. And I was sent on my way.

At home again, I noticed the front of my left leg had gone completely numb, but the back had a terrible shooting pain, the kind of cramping feeling you get with sciatica, from the top of the leg to the ankle. It made walking very difficult and I was still unable to wee. The pain got so excruciating that I had to go back to hospital. In fact, I was in hospital every two or three days from then on, so regularly that the staff there started to doubt my reasons for coming – the very staff I knew well, and who I'd worked with for many years.

There was more than an implication that I was one of those hospital hoppers, just coming for the morphine, so I was left with nitrous oxide, otherwise known as laughing gas – but there was nothing funny about it. I was told to draw on this until someone was ready to come and see me. It often took hours for someone to come, and this went on so long for so many times over the following weeks that I eventually developed a condition called transverse myelitis.

Using nitrous oxide can inhibit the absorption of vitamin B12 and this can cause damage to the myelin which insulates nerve fibres. For me the symptoms were numbness from the feet all the way up to vertebrae C1 to C7 (the neck essentially) and this began to affect my breathing, so I found myself rushed to hospital yet again.

And all this with a new-born baby at home.

Luckily my husband's employers were great about granting him leave so he could be there to look after Neve and the rest of my children, who were all under nine years old, while I went back and forth to hospital. My parents and his parents were also on hand as ever to help and thank God they were, otherwise, I don't know how we would have coped at that time.

Over those next awful months, I kept asking for an MRI, a scan, anything to show what was going on with me. I was convinced that the root of the problem which had started in the labour ward, had still not been found. Eventually after five months of terrible pain, I was reluctantly granted an MRI.

It was this MRI which revealed immediately and clearly that I had Cauda Equina Syndrome – something which needs emergency treatment within seventy-two hours of the onset of symptoms. I had had symptoms since Neve was born nearly five months earlier.

I, like many of the staff whose care I was under in Watford, had never heard of Cauda Equina Syndrome, but it is characterised by compression of the nerves at the lumbosacral joint, otherwise known as L5-S1. My epidural was given at L5. You don't have to be a spinal surgeon to see the correlation.

Despite having been a nurse at a time in the early '90s when lifting patients was the norm without any hoists to take the strain, I had never had a problem with my back, unlike many people with CES who often report a history of back issues before their injury. Never, until that epidural was given.

From the MRI room I was rushed straight to the neurological hospital in Queen's Square, London where I had a discectomy and laminectomy (where part of the bone is removed from the vertebrae). But unfortunately, neither were to be my last. Just five days later I had to go back for another discectomy at the same point in my spine. And the following month an MRI showed the need for yet another discectomy and simultaneous laminectomy. After these procedures, a spinal fluid leak occurred so I was back in theatre yet again, the fourth time in the space of about a month.

From then on, to deal with the pain, I have had to inject myself with morphine every four hours and with cyclizine every eight hours to combat the nausea caused by all the morphine. I was left, as many CES sufferers are, with the need to catheterize every four hours, the need to irrigate my bowels regularly, and great difficulty walking.

But most of all I was left with anger.

I felt my world crash down around me. I'd lost everything. My income, my dignity, my sense of self. I was no longer Ginette or Mum. I was some disabled person and my husband had become my carer.

As an EMT myself, I knew what Grant did all day at work as a paramedic. And then he had to come home and deal with me. It was like he never got to switch off from being the medical professional, the carer. If the district nurses were not able to come on time to administer my morphine injections, then Grant would do that too. I am technically able to give it to myself, but I can't bring myself to do so, particularly the cyclizine, because I know how painful it's going to be.

There have been occasions over the years where the doctors have suggested that I should be fitted with a permanent catheter attached to a bag, so I don't have to break my sleep by getting up to catheterize myself every night, but I have always refused. I am in my forties, for God's sake! And I knew that would kill any remnant of romance Grant and I had clung onto in our relationship. I wouldn't blame Grant for finding me unattractive with a bag hanging off of me. And I already had enough insecurities about my body image since CES – the horrendous scar down my back from four surgeries, for one thing. Also, for me, I like to wear nice skirts and dresses; that wouldn't be possible with a tube attached to me all the time. So, for the sake of our relationship, I am prepared to disturb my sleep and self-catheterize. That way, no one else needs to be involved. Yes, I am tired and yes, I am more prone to infections because of it, but my relationship with Grant and my self-esteem are too important to sacrifice for a little convenience.

Despite my love for Grant and the importance I place on our relationship, that anger I have can still raise its ugly head now and again, and in the heat of an argument I might find myself blaming him for my condition, saying things like:

'Why did you not help me out more? Why did you not stick up for me more? I was so vulnerable and yet you never came to the hospital, never took me to A&E. You were never there for me.'

This is of course deeply unfair and totally unreasonable for me to say when you recall that we had a new-born baby at the time, not to mention three other young children, and Grant had to look after all of them. I'm sure he would have happily come to the hospital to support me, but he didn't really have a choice. He was great holding the fort while I was away and it is totally selfish of me to think otherwise, but that anger I have is hard to shake off sometimes.

Thankfully after the surgeries I was referred quite quickly to the spinal unit at Stoke Mandeville Hospital and spent six weeks there learning how to deal with my condition – not only the mechanical stuff like catheterization, but the emotional stuff too.

My children were still so young and, having previously dealt with an abusive father, now they were having to deal with losing the mum they were so used to and missing the things I could do for them when they should have just been worrying about growing up like any other children. It was hard for them to understand why an ambulance had to come nearly every week and take me away for some reason or another – if it wasn't excruciating pain, it was because, being so unsteady on my feet, I had fallen, as I did down the stairs on one occasion, fracturing my coccyx. Or falling between the bath and sink and having to call the fire brigade to get me out – things like that episode are almost comical in hindsight, but certainly not at the time.

The children were all fantastic and have been so helpful and supportive to me since my injury, but there is no doubt they were all affected by it, especially Neve, who was the youngest and didn't understand why I needed to keep calling an ambulance. Nowadays if she sees an ambulance she freezes and trembles as it triggers old memories. She was also bullied in school to the extent that she is now home schooled. But at Stoke Mandeville, counselling was offered to all of my children as well as me and Grant. And the children embraced this, and got so much out of it, as it was handled so well by the staff there.

Meanwhile, I was freaking out at the idea of learning to catheterize myself, so the continence nurse at Stoke Mandeville came to my rescue. She was amazing. Going above and beyond anything you would expect from a nurse.

'You can do it. You *can*,' she would tell me.

And one night she came along to the toilet and stayed with me for over an hour after her shift should have finished. She showed me that it was OK. That anyone could have a catheter. She made sure we had a great laugh about the whole thing too and in doing so she saved my life that night. I was so close to giving up and I think she knew that. I'm so glad now that I didn't. I owe her so much.

Her attitude and the advice of the counsellors at Stoke Mandeville helped me to see that I was a mum of four and I needed to carry on, for them as much as myself and my husband.

But I did really miss my job. I missed the social aspect of it. And most of all I missed being someone who was good at helping others.

Knowing more than a little about the NHS, I am not scared to ask for what I need and, as time passed, I realised that I could be useful in encouraging other people with CES to ask for what they needed too, so I hooked up with the Cauda Equina Champions Charity and signed up to become a CES Buddy for newly injured people. Many of them tell me their GP has given up on them and they can't get the support services they need. So, I tell them how they should go back and persist, demand help even. I am happy to be able to guide them to find the support services they need. I finally feel now I have come full circle and am back in a role of helping others and hopefully making a difference in their lives.

The ambulance service in the '90s was a man's game. I was very much in the minority as a female EMT and I would often come up against misogyny and sexist abuse from patients, so I had to toughen up quite quickly and now I use that assertiveness when helping others with CES.

I am probably a little more equipped than many people to deal with the mechanics of my self-care due to my medical training. That combined with my assertiveness and natural determination has stood me in good stead for dealing with my condition in the longer term.

Grant and I have even started going on holidays again and in 2018 renewed our wedding vows in Lapland. At first, I would think about all the reasons why going away wouldn't work. I would think about all the things I couldn't do or the places I couldn't go anymore. I used to love going skiing, for example, but that was out of the question now. However, thinking outside the box a little, but we soon found other options. We decided to go on a cruise recently and that was amazing. No issues getting on board as there can be with flying. Medical staff on hand 24/7. Seeing beautiful parts of the world I might not have thought about seeing otherwise.

As a result of my injury, I have changed the way I think. I had to, as my life has changed so much. I try and focus less on the losses and more on the silver linings – like being at home more for my amazing children Lara, Alice, Jack, and Neve and even being able to help home school Neve. So, with each day that passes, I can keep the anger at bay for a little longer, and I'm starting to get a taste of that wonderfully normal life I used to have once again.

I would like to dedicate this story to my phenomenal husband Grant, my amazing children Lara, Alice, Jack, and Neve, and also my Mum and Dad, all of whom have showed the most incredible support and love throughout.

I would also like to thank Professor L Zrinzo, my consultant neurosurgeon, based at The National Neurological Hospital Queens Square and Mr. M. Belci, my consultant in spinal cord injury, based at Stoke Mandeville Spinal Unit.

LAURA'S STORY

A horse's tale.

I love caring for others, be they animal or human. I always have. But it is horses above all that I live for.

I grew up in Gloucestershire in a big family. I rode horses since I was four years old. I didn't always have the easiest of childhoods, but horses were a great solace to me in difficult times.

By the age of eighteen, I already lived by myself in a flat and was not afraid of being independent and making my own decisions, many of which were often made on the spur of the moment, such as my idea to move down to Bournemouth one day. At that time in 2002 there was always loads going on down there. Places to party, things to do and the beautiful New Forest right on the doorstep, a haven for horses and perfect for anyone as active as I was.

My parents helped me by packing up half my life in their car and half in mine and I went to stay with my aunt and uncle while I found my feet. I soon found a job in a hotel, met loads of great people, and finally felt I was starting to live my life and leave the hardships of my childhood behind.

Pretty soon after I turned nineteen, I got together with one of my colleagues. He was much older than me and already had three kids, ranging in age from three to eleven. It didn't seem like the obvious choice of relationship for a young woman just starting to spread her wings, but you can't help who you fall in love with. Besides, I bonded well with the kids and even got on with their mother. It was a hell of an adjustment for me at first, but one which I was very happy to make.

I brought my love of the outdoors to my new family. We would go hiking and camping especially in the New Forest and even took up scuba diving, which is a surprisingly wonderful thing to do in the apparently murky waters off the south coast of England. I even got my own horse. I could never stand to be away from these majestic creatures too long and soon changed my job so I could work with horses too. I became a riding instructor at one of the riding schools in the New Forest, both teaching and leading riders through the national parkland. I would spend eight hours a day in the saddle, rain or shine, even in snow.

I was in my element.

Life was good and the cherry on top of it all was getting married to my partner in Florida in 2005. We went out there to have a holiday with my family, but halfway through surprised them with the news that we were getting married the next day. It was certainly a surprise, even a bit of a shock, especially to my dad, who had never been good at letting go of his little girl, but everything went without a hitch. In fact. it was amazing. After the wedding in a beautiful white chapel on International Drive we celebrated in the Disney entertainment mecca of Pleasure Island where we were given the honour of setting off the midnight fireworks.

It was a great start to our married life. But I was still only twenty-one.

The next decade was a period of great change for me (as they are for anyone in their twenties) finding out who I was and what I really wanted from life. And so, by the time I turned twenty-six, I had decided that this marriage was not really what I wanted from life; it wasn't working for me, for who I was now, and my husband and I agreed, mutually and amicably, to part ways.

I didn't really want to leave my beloved Bournemouth, but I went back to stay with my parents in Gloucestershire while I regrouped and worked out what was next for me. And then after a year or so back there I found myself in a new relationship. It wasn't a good relationship, and it soon broke down, but there was one wonderful thing that came out of it: my son.

He was such a blessing, a miracle in fact, because I had always been told that I would struggle to have children and I had already had many miscarriages. That was hard for me to take coming from such a very large family. I had five siblings. One of my sisters had six kids, one of my brothers had five. My mum was one of thirteen and my dad was one of nine. I felt it was my calling to be a mother to many. It was the kind of environment I was used to while growing up and one I wanted to recreate in my adulthood. Not being able to have many children myself leaves me to this day feeling incomplete as a woman; it always niggles at me that I couldn't have more, but of course, I am so grateful for my son, and I love him to bits.

When my son was three months old, I struck out on my own again and found us a flat in Cheltenham. By this time, online dating was becoming a thing, and I decided, with a few failed relationships behind me that had come about the traditional way, why not try a different approach?

Before long I found myself chatting to someone online. We had a lot in common and we both had kids already, which helped. He was from Swindon, and I was an hour up the road in Cheltenham, but instead of meeting halfway for our first date, we decided to meet in the place we both happened to love more than anywhere else: Bournemouth.

My son was eight months old by now and I took him on the date with me. Well, this guy and I both knew that if we took each other on we took on our kids too, so why not start as we meant to go on?

We got on like a house on fire. For the next couple of years, we to and froed between our respective homes, and in 2014 I got pregnant. I was so excited to be adding to what I hoped would be a growing family, to give my son a sibling, one of many more, just as I and my parents had enjoyed. However, at the three-month scan in Gloucester, I was told there was no baby, just the amniotic sack.

My heart was broken.

And to make matters worse, a week after the scan I began haemorrhaging and was rushed to Swindon hospital. It was there I was told that I had had what is known as a molar pregnancy where the placenta had developed abnormally creating a collection of cells that were in danger of developing into cancerous cells. It had been totally missed by the hospital in Gloucester.

My partner, who supported me through this awful ordeal, suggested that having faced such adversity together, we were actually stronger as a couple. He was right. Coming through this had indeed brought us closer and so we felt it was the perfect time to move in together.

I upped sticks again and went to Swindon.

It was hard to move on, surrounded by all the baby things we had already bought in anticipation of the birth, but we both tried our best to get over the grief and get on with our lives.

Horses came to the rescue again.

In Swindon I got myself a job as a horse nutritionist and then, after a short spell as a patient transport assistant working in a great team in the NHS, I became sales manager for an equine bedding company. I met some great new friends through this work and of course it wasn't long before I acquired more horses of my own.

I brought my active outdoors life to my new family, even managing to get us all up to the summit of Snowdon four times. Since he was so good at DIY, I roped my partner into the world of my horses by getting him to fix things around the stables. He didn't profess to be a horse person at all, but it wasn't long before I caught him stroking them and talking affectionately to them. I made sure the kids were all familiar with horses as soon as possible and they soon loved them, almost as much as I do.

Having horses takes up a lot of your money and a lot of your time. It eats into your social life, but the stables became our social life. In the summer we'd have barbeques, and the kids would be in the pool at the horse yard all day, and then in the autumn we'd have bonfires at night. It was a community within itself. We had great friends there and my sense of belonging had never been more solid.

Back problems are par for the course for horse riders. You fall off plenty of times when you're learning, you lug hay bales and heavy bags of feed about all the time. I had my fair share of muscular aches and pains, but nothing I ever worried about.

Then, in late December 2018, I was just sitting at my desk at work, when the toes in my left foot went numb. I shifted about and loosened my boot, thinking my footwear was just too tight. It wouldn't surprise me; like a lot of women, I'd often try and fit into a size too small to look more petite. But that didn't help. As the morning wore on, the numbness started to spread from my big toe along to my other toes and across my foot. I took my boot off and moved my foot about to try and get the feeling back into it, as you do when you have pins and needles, but that didn't help either. My legs were starting to ache now, as was my back, and the ache soon became pain. It was such an odd feeling that I started to feel anxious about it; anxious enough to call my G.P.

I explained my symptoms and the doctor told me they were 'Red flag' symptoms. I had no idea what 'Red flag' symptoms were, but he told me it was serious. I needed to get myself over to the hospital as quickly as possible. He called the hospital himself and arranged for me to bypass A&E and go straight to the surgical assessment unit. So, by mid-afternoon, with the reduced sensation now spreading, I made arrangements for my partner to make sure he was home when the kids got back from school, and I went to the hospital, where I sat for a couple of hours waiting to be seen.

By the time I got to see a doctor I explained that the pain was now radiating from my back down to my legs and the lack of sensation, which was most prominent in my left leg, was also in my saddle area too. Generally, my muscles below the waist, particularly on the left side, were starting to feel weak; I had a horrible sense of everything drooping.

The doctor did pin prick tests on my skin and muscle tone tests on my anal sphincter. Both were not great results by any means, so he ordered an MRI. The trouble was the MRI wasn't possible for some reason until the following day. I was told to come back at 7:30 in the morning.

I went home and the symptoms got worse overnight. The pain increased as did the reduced sensation. I had no idea what was going on with me.

My partner was equally confused. It was so hard to explain to him why I couldn't move and what kind of sensations, or lack of them, I was experiencing.

First thing in the morning, I was back at the hospital, and the pain was unbearably bad now. After waiting an hour or so I was examined by a different doctor to the one I'd seen yesterday and eventually told by a nurse that the MRI scanner still was not available.

'You need to go home,' she said. 'And we will contact you to tell you when you can come back for the scan.'

I wanted to cry.

After falling off horses and being generally active all my life I'd developed quite a high pain threshold, but I was in agony now and the thought of being sent home without treatment or any idea what was wrong was too much to bear.

But sent home I was.

I could hardly walk properly now but managed to drive myself home. We live in an old coach house. You have to go up a floor from the front door, to the living space, and I had to drag myself up those stairs. I called in sick and got myself into bed where I lay alone for the rest of the day.

By the afternoon the pain was ten-fold what it was in the morning, a sensation of my body being ripped apart. I couldn't move and this pain radiating from my back across my hips made childbirth seem easy.

I called 111 and told them what was going on and they told me they were sending an ambulance.

While I was waiting, my partner came home having picked the kids up from school. He heard me crying out in the bedroom and came through to see what was wrong. I told him how I wanted the pain to end. I needed to move to try and make it go away but I couldn't move myself. I asked him to help me get up, but as soon as he tried the pain got even worse, if that was possible. It felt as if someone had taken a machete and slashed it across my spine. I begged him to put me back on the bed and I lay there sobbing, wishing someone would put me out of my misery.

When the ambulance arrived, the paramedics could see how much pain I was in but trying to find a vein in my shocked body for intravenous pain relief was so hard, they resorted to jabbing me with morphine. The paramedic knew just by looking at me that I had a spinal injury but that was the first I had ever heard of all this being related to my spine.

They blue-lighted me to A&E, but when I got there it was so busy. There were ambulance crews from all over, lining up in the corridor with their patients waiting to be seen. Despite the morphine, I was screaming in agony by this time, so much so that other paramedics, who had stabilized their patients, were offering me their place in the queue. We were there for hours. The paramedics were trying to get me prioritised until they had to leave and then I was left screaming on a bed right in front of the nurses' station.

My screams must have been so annoying for them that I was then put into a room on my own wishing my partner hadn't had to stay home to look after the kids. I felt isolated and ignored. I was seen by a doctor and a nurse came in to drain my bladder using a catheter as I still couldn't go by myself. Then at 1AM I was finally told that, since I was just waiting for an MRI, that is what I should continue to do. At home.

Apparently, whatever I had wasn't too serious, they 'saw it all the time, a bit of back pain.' So, I had to call my partner to come and get me. He had to wake the kids up and bring them with him in the middle of the night, on a school night too. I went home feeling as if I had just been a nuisance to everybody.

But nothing had changed as far as my symptoms were concerned. So, for the next four long days, as Christmas approached, I remained in pain, unable to move properly, unbale to go to the toilet. I would sit there for ages trying to go and, when I wasn't on the toilet, I would get little leakages. I was baffled.

When the hospital finally rang, they said could I come in on Boxing Day for the scan. I asked if they could see me sooner, but they said that was the earliest they could do.

I was so miserable by this point, dosing up on painkillers, my kids anxious, not knowing what was happening. My son, who has some learning difficulties, was particularly worried. We had lost my dad a few years, before when he was only four, and he had taken it really hard. They had been very close and now I could see that he feared losing me too. I tried to keep all my emotions bottled up for the sake of him, tried to hide what was going on. When Christmas Day came, I insisted upon doing the tradition of going to my partner's parents' house where we'd have dinner and open presents. My partner had to carry me down the stairs and out to the car and I endured the pain for as long as I could, but by early afternoon I had to ask him to take me home. I didn't want to be the party pooper, but the pain was too unbearable. Everyone was so understanding, but I felt awful, as if I was letting them all down.

Boxing Day came and I went for the scan at long last. My partner drove me there hand my son came along too.

It wasn't many minutes after the scan that I was told that I needed to go to John Radcliffe hospital in Oxford as a matter of urgency. I asked my partner to go and get me some things from home and I was rushed in an ambulance to Oxford where a lovely surgeon explained everything. For the first time it was made clear that I had something called Cauda Equina Syndrome.

'Cauda equina means horse's tail,' the doctor said.

How ironic, I thought. But as the severity of my situation became clear I was soon scared, shitless.

'We need to operate immediately to stop you being paralysed for the rest of your life. You've been left far too long already, so there will almost certainly be complications after.'

I broke down. I couldn't take it all in. I couldn't believe what I was hearing. I tried to comprehend what my life was going to be like after this operation, but it was all too much. When I was told the risks involved in the operation, it made me want to refuse to go through with it, but at the same time I knew it had to be done. It was an unreal situation. Talk about a rock and a hard place!

Just then my partner and son arrived. I was so thankful to see them before I went under, but my son looked ghostly pale, I could see the fear in his eyes as he wondered what the hell was going to happen. The nurses, however, could see it too and they were wonderful, distracting him with a big box of chocolates and heaps of kindness as I was wheeled away.

People with Cauda Equina Syndrome often say that the first thing they notice when they wake up after surgery is that the pain is gone. There might be other complications to deal with, but they are at least grateful for not having that excruciating pain anymore. But, in my case, nothing had changed. There was no relief. The pain was still there, just as agonizing as before. I still had reduced sensation in both legs, and I couldn't get out of bed.

For the next three weeks I remained in hospital, trying in vain to get about on crutches and struggling to urinate. The occupational therapists and physios there did all they could, but before I left the hospital the spinal nurse was very clear:

'Your life has changed significantly,' she explained. 'You now need to adapt to your new life. You're not going to be able to do the things you did before and there will be many problems to overcome as you go forward.'

She wasn't wrong.

'We've done all we can,' the surgeon said when he came to check on me. 'Only time will tell just what issues this will leave you with, but there was a lot of damage to the nerves and a lot of fragments that we couldn't remove, so there is a possibility it could happen again.'

I went home with the surgeon's words still ringing in my ears fearing that I would have to go through this trauma all over again, and indeed I was rushed back to the hospital on a number of occasions over the following months with recurring pain, so severe in one case that the only thing that could stop it was ketamine, which is used as a horse tranquilizer – the irony again wasn't lost on me.

I asked the doctors at the hospital if a spinal fusion operation was possible to reduce the likelihood of a relapse of Cauda Equina Syndrome, but they kept putting me off. I begged them to do it, to stop the pain that I still had to endure, but they eventually told me that the risks were too great, and they wouldn't do the operation.

I spent the first year after the injury in a wheelchair. It took me a long time to learn to get about on crutches. I had to rely on family and friends to help me go to the toilet, which was frankly embarrassing. My mum and my sister would have to come all the way from Gloucester just to help me have a shower. And I knew it was breaking my mum's heart to see me in the state I was in.

My relationship was under enormous strain too. Despite everything we'd been through in the past which had brought us closer, my partner and I now began to argue. He felt frustrated and I felt useless. I was a grown woman in my late thirties, for God's sake! I should be able to look after myself.

A few months after coming out of hospital I hit rock bottom and I wanted to end my life. I didn't want to suffer the pain anymore and I didn't want to rely on people. But then my son came to me and said in his wonderfully innocent way, 'Don't worry, mummy. I love you and I am going to help you all I can.'

And that turned everything around for me.

I knew I couldn't leave him. I had to stick around for him. I knew the frustration I felt was that I was the one who always liked to help others. I always put other people – or animals – before myself. That was the way I liked things to be. So, if I was able to help my son at all right now, it was by not going through with what I saw as my selfish desire to end my life.

The other significant thing that helped me turn things around at that point was when the spinal nurse at John Radcliffe hospital managed to get me a place at the Duke of Cornwall Spinal Treatment Centre in Salisbury. They offered me a three day stay in the July following my injury during which time they would try to help me learn how to manage better at home. I knew that places at this centre were hard to come by and that they had really good results, so I wrote to them and told them I very much wanted to take them up on their offer.

I couldn't wait for July to come. Every day was a struggle until then, but I was hopeful that my time in Salisbury would offer some solutions to the problems I was having.

When I got to the centre, they quickly realised I had bigger issues than even they had thought, so, my three-day stay, turned into more than a week. It was a lovely place to be and a revelation. Until then I had been sitting on the toilet every day for ages trying to make myself pee by pushing down on my bladder. At Salisbury I was informed that this was a very unhealthy practice, and I was promptly shown how to catheterize. Until then I had been struggling with getting around in ill-fitting wheelchairs. At Salisbury I was shown how to get around properly, I was shown how important it was to find the right wheelchair for each individual and I was also given fantastic physio to try and regain some strength in my legs. Until then I had been struggling to open my bowels. Salisbury discovered I was completely impacted, a very dangerous condition to have. They introduced me to Peristeen, a trans anal irrigation system, which was, quite literally, a life saver.

I felt much more confident after my stay there; better equipped to manage things and safer in the knowledge that I would always have support from them. They were, and still are, only ever a phone call away. They put me in touch with the Continence team who would visit at home and scan my bladder, which to this day seems to have a mind of its own: sometimes it retains too much, sometimes I just can't stop going to the toilet. I can get around with crutches now over short distances, but the pain is something that I am forced to manage every day. This takes its toll on my mental health and my relationship.

It was only a year ago (a couple of years after the injury) that my partner and I almost split up. He had been going through his own battles and, for a time there I almost forgot, as my own troubles naturally consumed me, that he needed support as much as I did. He'd had a motorbike accident before we met which nearly took his life and resulted in him being in hospital for a year. He recovered physically, although he now has metal plates in his wrist and a hip replacement, but the trauma resulted in ongoing depression for him. Coupled with trying to look after me, his depression soon became overwhelming. However, he sought help and opened up to me, about it. That's when I knew we both had to work out our problems with each other, for each other. No one else was going to help.

No one except for my horses, of course.

I can't go and ride and manage my horses as I used to, but the community of friends and colleagues I had built up around horses came to the rescue in a big way. My employers were very supportive and allowed me to start working from home as and when my health allowed me to, which was extremely flexible of them. My friends helped out at the yard and took my son whenever I needed a little time to rest. And because I had been going through so many issues myself, it actually made me even more empathetic to those facing challenges of their own. I realised that I could still help others, with the help of my horses, by loaning them out.

Our biggest horse now goes to the Riders for the Disabled Association during term time and helps kids with autism particularly. He comes home at the holidays and then my kids get to ride him too.

When I first had CES, many people encouraged me to sell the horses, but there was no way I was going to do that. They are and always have been my lifeline. They keep me going. They give me a purpose, a goal, and a challenge.

And the next challenge is for me to get back out there with them too.

My fabulous horse, who works with children with disabilities so well, is now going to be broken to drive. This means he'll hopefully soon be comfortable with pulling the cart, which my partner has lovingly restored for me. By the end of this year, I expect to be out and about with my beloved horses again and the only cauda equina I want to feel is my pony's tail swishing in the wind as we race along the bridleway, free once more.

I would like to say a big thank you to the nursing staff at John Radcliffe Hospital Level 3 West Wing for the support and kindness given during my stay. Also, to the doctors on this ward who took the time to explain everything to me so clearly.

And I cannot forget the team at the Duke of Cornwall Spinal Treatment Centre for their amazing help to get my life back on track and the ongoing support they still provide when needed.

MIKE HUTTON

Consultant Spine Surgeon
National lead for spinal services optimisation and recovery
for the BestMSK Collaborative

When I was fourteen years old, I spent six months in hospital with an illness that doctors struggled to diagnose despite their best efforts. I was eventually diagnosed with a rare condition that I've had to live with ever since. It was during this time that I decided I wanted to be a doctor and dedicated my efforts to achieving that goal.

I also loved watching and playing rugby (not surprisingly, as my parents were both New Zealanders) and again strived to be the best I could. I eventually played rugby professionally for Richmond, The Barbarians and England Under 21s. My career was cut short by a broken leg at the age of twenty-eight and I became a consultant spine surgeon nine years later.

Many of the stories I've read in this book from patients who have had Cauda Equina Syndrome (CES) remind me of dealing with adversity and challenging said adversity with a positive approach. These stories, I'm sure, will help patients who have had this unfortunate condition.

CES is very rare (1-3 in 100,000 population). It is fair to say we don't understand many aspects of CES, and we see many patients who may possibly have it but turn out not to on investigation. We also struggle to know reliably how much and within what timescale emergency surgery prevents deterioration or improves outcomes for patients.

In 2016 I was asked to lead a review of all spinal services in England. The Getting it Right First Time

(GIRFT) programme, now a part of NHS England, involved visiting 185 units which provided both emergency and elective care for patients with spinal conditions. Our aim was to identify unwarranted variation in practice and make recommendations on how we could improve our spinal services for patients.

One of the most common conditions that spinal teams have to deal with, is patients who have suspected CES. Our GIRFT review found considerable variation in the way suspected CES was diagnosed, in access to MRI out of hours and access to emergency operating lists. One of the main issues with suspected CES is that, while many opinions exist as to what 'right' looks like, the scientific evidence to support these opinions is poor.

The Healthcare Safety Investigation Board (HSIB) has recommended that we now identify what best practice is for this condition, and the NHS England Best MSK Health Collaborative has been tasked to produce a best practice pathway for clinicians. As chair of this national pathway for suspected Cauda Equina Syndrome, I am excited about the cross-speciality working and involvement of patient groups such as the Cauda Equina Champions Charity and am confident that this will help drive improvement of the management of patients with suspected CES.

References

Get it Right First Time Report - Spinal services

www.gettingitrightfirsttime.co.uk/surgical-speciality/spinal-surgery/

HSIB Report – Timely detection and treatment of Cauda Equina Syndrome

www.hsib.org.uk/investigations-and-reports/timely-detection-and-treatment-of-spinal-nerve-compression-cauda-equina-syndrome-in-patients-with-back-pain/timely-detection-and-treatment-of-cauda-equina-syndrome/

ABOUT OUR CHARITY

Cauda Equina Champions Charity is a patient led charity that aims to raise awareness of CES and support everyone affected by it. Growing from a Facebook support group over ten years ago the charity is now the leading voice for Cauda Equina Syndrome in the UK and abroad.

- 03335 777113 National Helpline
- Patient support packs
- Face to face support meetings
- Online support group
- Psychosexual therapy service
- CES Buddy service
- Navigating the NHS service
- Social events
- www.championscharity.org.uk

ACKNOWLEDGEMENTS

We would like to express our heartfelt thanks and appreciation to the following people and organisations whose generous contributions enabled us to publish this book. We are extremely grateful for their expertise, skill and support for this project.

- To the wonderful Mr. Mecci, Consultant in Spinal Cord injuries at The Golden Jubilee Spinal centre, James Cook University Hospital, Middlesbrough for his unrelenting passion and championing of the plight of cauda equina syndrome patients.

- To the charismatic and inspiring Mike Hutton, National lead for spinal services optimisation and recovery for the BestMSK Collaborative for his commitment and hard work, in an area fraught with difficulties, to the development and implementation of a new national pathway for Suspected Cauda Equina Syndrome.

- Our amazing support group members, for bravely sharing their stories to raise awareness of Cauda Equina Syndrome and help others diagnosed with the condition.

- Warren FitzGerald – Writer and patient listener www.warrenfitzgerald.co.uk

- Jay Stansfield – Cover design and art https://jaystansfield.com

- To members of our Legal panel for their valuable support and expertise, especially to Eddie Jones who has supported us from the beginning.

- Julianne Moore – Irwin Mitchell
  www.irwinmitchell.com

- Eddie Jones - JMW Solicitors
  www.jmw.co.uk

- Olive Lewin – Leigh Day Solicitors
  www.leighday.co.uk

- Dan O'Keeffe – Moosa-Duke Solicitors
  www.moosaduke.com

- Simon Elliman – RWK Goodman Solicitors
  www.rwkgoodman.com

- Emma Doughty – Slater and Gordon Solicitors
  www.slatergordon.co.uk